# Perfect Weight
# JOURNAL

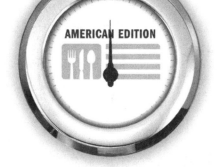

AMERICAN EDITION

# JORDAN RUBIN

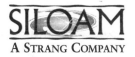

SILOAM
A STRANG COMPANY

Most STRANG COMMUNICATIONS/CHARISMA HOUSE/SILOAM/FRONTLINE/EXCEL BOOKS/REALMS products are available at special quantity discounts for bulk purchase for sales promotions, premiums, fund-raising, and educational needs. For details, write Strang Communications/Charisma House/Siloam/FrontLine/Excel Books/Realms, 600 Rinehart Road, Lake Mary, Florida 32746, or telephone (407) 333-0600.

PERFECT WEIGHT JOURNAL—AMERICAN EDITION by Jordan Rubin
Published by Siloam
A Strang Company
600 Rinehart Road
Lake Mary, Florida 32746
www.siloam.com

Cover Designer: Bill Johnson

International Standard Book Number: 978-1-59979-267-5

Neither the publisher nor the author is engaged in rendering professional advice or services to the individual reader. The ideas, procedures, and suggestions in this book are not intended as a substitute for consulting with your physician. All matters regarding your health require medical supervision. Neither the author nor the publisher shall be liable or responsible for any loss or damage allegedly arising from any information or suggestion in this book.

While the author has made every effort to provide accurate telephone numbers and Internet addresses at the time of publication, neither the publisher nor the author assumes any responsibility for errors or for changes that occur after publication.

08 09 10 11 12 — 9 8 7 6 5 4 3 2 1
Printed in the United States of America

# Table of Contents

# Welcome

If you are looking to change your diet and your life, then welcome to the *Perfect Weight Journal*. Maybe it's been years since you have woken up feeling refreshed or have attacked the day with spring in your step. Maybe your life has been marked by regular visits to the family doctor and expensive specialists who struggle to find out what's "wrong" with you. Maybe you gulp down powerful drugs to fight off the ravages of hypertension, type 2 diabetes, heartburn, and a host of other ailments—and wonder if the side effects aren't worse than the disease. If this sounds like you, then the health recommendations set forth in the book *Perfect Weight America* and this companion journal will hand you the tools to transform yourself in ways you never thought possible.

This journal is designed to be used along with *Perfect Weight America*, which provides everything you need to know about this sixteen-week, four-phase program that involves a comprehensive eating plan, taking nutritional supplements, reserving time for exercise, drinking plenty of water, eating healthy snacks, and embarking on seasonal "detox" cleanses. Although this program comes with no guarantees, we are confident that you will experience a personal transformation as well as weight loss, decrease in disease risk, and improved mental acuity and physical vitality.

Perfect Weight America calls for an attitude adjustment—fast. The most important outlook you can have during your sixteen-week experience is this: *I'm doing this for my health. The more I put into it, the more I will receive from it. If I give this my best effort, then I can expect the best results.*

The Perfect Weight America program is the brainchild of author and speaker Jordan Rubin, whose book *The Maker's Diet* was on the *New York Times* bestseller's list for forty-six weeks. The Perfect Weight America campaign has been gaining momentum ever since 126 participants in Ohio completed a community-based campaign called Healthy Toledo in 2007. Now, Jordan would like you to jump on the Perfect Weight America bandwagon. If you're ready to make a remarkable lifestyle change, then welcome aboard!

**—The Perfect Weight America Team**

# Determining Your Perfect Weight

By using this journal along with the book *Perfect Weight America*, you have the opportunity to determine your perfect weight. You will do this by taking into consideration the amount of weight you need to lose, your bone structure, your muscle mass, your genetics, and any associated risk factors due to your weight. Certain quantitative benchmarks can show you where you stand today and how your weight, body fat composition, and waist size have improved after completing the Perfect Weight program. Let's take a closer look at these calculations.

## Body Mass Index

Body mass index is a fitness-scale method that uses a mathematical formula to measure a person's height relative to his or her weight, although the results have to be taken with a grain of salt. As a strict formula, the body mass index equals a person's weight in kilograms divided by height in meters squared.

$$\text{BMI (kg/m2)} = \text{weight (lbs)} * 703 / \text{height (in)} / \text{height (in)}.$$

A far easier way to calculate your body mass index would be to use the body mass index chart on the next page. Find your height and then swish your finger down to your weight. The number at the intersection of your height and weight is your BMI.

The BMI breakdown goes like this:

- 18 or lower: underweight
- 19–24: normal
- 25–29: overweight
- 30–39: obese
- 40–54: extremely obese

As an example, someone standing 5 feet 10 inches tall and weighing more than 209 pounds would have a BMI of 30, earning him or her a classification of obese on the body mass index scale. About 30 percent of the U.S. adult population has a BMI of 30 or more, which is why we have an obesity epidemic.

In general, the greater the BMI, the greater the risk of contracting diseases associated with obesity.

## Body Mass Index for adults Table

| Height (inches) | Normal | | | | | | Overweight | | | | | Obese | | | | | | | | | |
|---|---|---|---|---|---|---|---|---|---|---|---|---|---|---|---|---|---|---|---|---|---|
| BMI | 19 | 20 | 21 | 22 | 23 | 24 | 25 | 26 | 27 | 28 | 29 | 30 | 31 | 32 | 33 | 34 | 35 | 36 | 37 | 38 | 39 |
| | Body Weight (pounds) | | | | | | | | | | | | | | | | | | | | |
| 58 | 91 | 96 | 100 | 105 | 110 | 115 | 119 | 124 | 129 | 134 | 138 | 143 | 148 | 153 | 158 | 162 | 167 | 172 | 177 | 181 | 186 |
| 59 | 94 | 99 | 104 | 109 | 114 | 119 | 124 | 128 | 133 | 138 | 143 | 148 | 153 | 158 | 163 | 168 | 173 | 178 | 183 | 188 | 193 |
| 60 | 97 | 102 | 107 | 112 | 118 | 123 | 128 | 133 | 138 | 143 | 148 | 153 | 158 | 163 | 168 | 174 | 179 | 184 | 189 | 194 | 199 |
| 61 | 100 | 106 | 111 | 116 | 122 | 127 | 132 | 137 | 143 | 148 | 153 | 158 | 164 | 169 | 174 | 180 | 185 | 190 | 195 | 201 | 206 |
| 62 | 104 | 109 | 115 | 120 | 126 | 131 | 136 | 142 | 147 | 153 | 158 | 164 | 169 | 175 | 180 | 186 | 191 | 196 | 202 | 207 | 213 |
| 63 | 107 | 113 | 118 | 124 | 130 | 135 | 141 | 146 | 152 | 158 | 163 | 169 | 175 | 180 | 186 | 191 | 197 | 203 | 208 | 214 | 220 |
| 64 | 110 | 116 | 122 | 128 | 134 | 140 | 145 | 151 | 157 | 163 | 169 | 174 | 180 | 186 | 192 | 197 | 204 | 209 | 215 | 221 | 227 |
| 65 | 114 | 120 | 126 | 132 | 138 | 144 | 150 | 156 | 162 | 168 | 174 | 180 | 186 | 192 | 198 | 204 | 210 | 216 | 222 | 228 | 234 |
| 66 | 118 | 124 | 130 | 136 | 142 | 148 | 155 | 161 | 167 | 173 | 179 | 186 | 192 | 198 | 204 | 210 | 216 | 223 | 229 | 235 | 241 |
| 67 | 121 | 127 | 134 | 140 | 146 | 153 | 159 | 166 | 172 | 178 | 185 | 191 | 198 | 204 | 211 | 217 | 223 | 230 | 236 | 242 | 249 |
| 68 | 125 | 131 | 138 | 144 | 151 | 158 | 164 | 171 | 177 | 184 | 190 | 197 | 203 | 210 | 216 | 223 | 230 | 236 | 243 | 249 | 256 |
| 69 | 128 | 135 | 142 | 149 | 155 | 162 | 169 | 176 | 182 | 189 | 196 | 203 | 209 | 216 | 223 | 230 | 236 | 243 | 250 | 257 | 263 |
| 70 | 132 | 139 | 146 | 153 | 160 | 167 | 174 | 181 | 188 | 195 | 202 | 209 | 216 | 222 | 229 | 236 | 243 | 250 | 257 | 264 | 271 |
| 71 | 136 | 143 | 150 | 157 | 165 | 172 | 179 | 186 | 193 | 200 | 208 | 215 | 222 | 229 | 236 | 243 | 250 | 257 | 265 | 272 | 279 |
| 72 | 140 | 147 | 154 | 162 | 169 | 177 | 184 | 191 | 199 | 206 | 213 | 221 | 228 | 235 | 242 | 250 | 258 | 265 | 272 | 279 | 287 |
| 73 | 144 | 151 | 159 | 166 | 174 | 182 | 189 | 197 | 204 | 212 | 219 | 227 | 235 | 242 | 250 | 257 | 265 | 272 | 280 | 288 | 295 |
| 74 | 148 | 155 | 163 | 171 | 179 | 186 | 194 | 202 | 210 | 218 | 225 | 233 | 241 | 249 | 256 | 264 | 272 | 280 | 287 | 295 | 303 |
| 75 | 152 | 160 | 168 | 176 | 184 | 192 | 200 | 208 | 216 | 224 | 232 | 240 | 248 | 256 | 264 | 272 | 279 | 287 | 295 | 303 | 311 |
| 76 | 156 | 164 | 172 | 180 | 189 | 197 | 205 | 213 | 221 | 230 | 238 | 246 | 254 | 263 | 271 | 279 | 287 | 295 | 304 | 312 | 320 |

### Extreme Obesity

| Height (inches) | | | | | | | | | Body Weight (pounds) | | | | | | |
|---|---|---|---|---|---|---|---|---|---|---|---|---|---|---|---|
| BMI | 40 | 41 | 42 | 43 | 44 | 45 | 46 | 47 | 48 | 49 | 50 | 51 | 52 | 53 | 54 |
| 58 | 191 | 196 | 201 | 205 | 210 | 215 | 220 | 224 | 229 | 234 | 239 | 244 | 248 | 253 | 258 |
| 59 | 198 | 203 | 208 | 212 | 217 | 222 | 227 | 232 | 237 | 242 | 247 | 252 | 257 | 262 | 267 |
| 60 | 204 | 209 | 215 | 220 | 225 | 230 | 235 | 240 | 245 | 250 | 255 | 261 | 266 | 271 | 276 |
| 61 | 211 | 217 | 222 | 227 | 232 | 238 | 243 | 248 | 254 | 259 | 264 | 269 | 275 | 280 | 285 |
| 62 | 218 | 224 | 229 | 235 | 240 | 246 | 251 | 256 | 262 | 267 | 273 | 278 | 284 | 289 | 295 |
| 63 | 225 | 231 | 237 | 242 | 248 | 254 | 259 | 265 | 270 | 278 | 282 | 287 | 293 | 299 | 304 |
| 64 | 232 | 238 | 244 | 250 | 256 | 262 | 267 | 273 | 279 | 285 | 291 | 296 | 302 | 308 | 314 |
| 65 | 240 | 246 | 252 | 258 | 264 | 270 | 276 | 282 | 288 | 294 | 300 | 306 | 312 | 318 | 324 |
| 66 | 247 | 253 | 260 | 266 | 272 | 278 | 284 | 291 | 297 | 303 | 309 | 315 | 322 | 328 | 334 |
| 67 | 255 | 261 | 268 | 274 | 280 | 287 | 293 | 299 | 306 | 312 | 319 | 325 | 331 | 338 | 344 |
| 68 | 262 | 269 | 276 | 282 | 289 | 295 | 302 | 308 | 315 | 322 | 328 | 335 | 341 | 348 | 354 |
| 69 | 270 | 277 | 284 | 291 | 297 | 304 | 311 | 318 | 324 | 331 | 338 | 345 | 351 | 358 | 365 |
| 70 | 278 | 285 | 292 | 299 | 306 | 313 | 320 | 327 | 334 | 341 | 348 | 355 | 362 | 369 | 376 |
| 71 | 286 | 293 | 301 | 308 | 315 | 322 | 329 | 338 | 343 | 351 | 358 | 365 | 372 | 379 | 386 |
| 72 | 294 | 302 | 309 | 316 | 324 | 331 | 338 | 346 | 353 | 361 | 368 | 375 | 383 | 390 | 397 |
| 73 | 302 | 310 | 318 | 325 | 333 | 340 | 348 | 355 | 363 | 371 | 378 | 386 | 393 | 401 | 408 |
| 74 | 311 | 319 | 326 | 334 | 342 | 350 | 358 | 365 | 373 | 381 | 389 | 396 | 404 | 412 | 420 |
| 75 | 319 | 327 | 335 | 343 | 351 | 358 | 367 | 375 | 383 | 391 | 399 | 407 | 415 | 423 | 431 |

Courtesy of National Heart, Lung, and Blood Institute, National Institutes of Health

## BMI Categories

- Underweight = < 18.5
- Normal weight = 18.5–24.9
- Overweight = 25–29.9
- Obesity = BMI of 30 or greater

## Frame Size

As explained in greater detail in the book *Perfect Weight America*, it is important to weigh your BMI against your body-frame size. The simplest method to calculate your frame size is to grab your wrist with the other hand and try to touch your thumb and index finger where the wrist meets the hand. If your fingers do not touch, you're a big-boned person with a large body frame. If your thumb and index finger just meet, you have a medium frame. If they overlap, you have a small frame.

If you have a larger frame, that will shift your perfect weight higher than the charted BMI normal range. By factoring your frame size into the equation for your perfect weight, you can better interpret the BMI figures.

## Body Fat Percentage

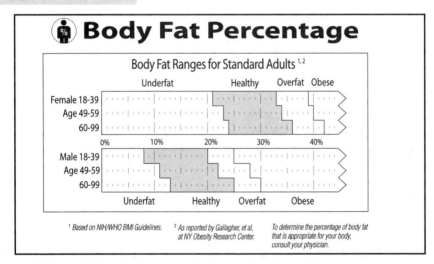

# Body Fat Percentage

### Body Fat Ranges for Standard Adults [1,2]

|  | Underfat | Healthy | Overfat | Obese |
| --- | --- | --- | --- | --- |
| Female 18-39 |  |  |  |  |
| Age 49-59 |  |  |  |  |
| 60-99 |  |  |  |  |

0%    10%    20%    30%    40%

| Male 18-39 |  |  |  |  |
| Age 49-59 |  |  |  |  |
| 60-99 |  |  |  |  |

Underfat    Healthy    Overfat    Obese

[1] Based on NIH/WHO BMI Guidelines.    [2] As reported by Gallagher, et al, at NY Obesity Research Center.    To determine the percentage of body fat that is appropriate for your body, consult your physician.

By definition, body fat percentage is an estimate of the fraction of the total body mass that is adipose tissue (fat) as opposed to lean body mass, which is muscle, bone, organ tissue, blood, and everything else. It is more accurate as a measure of excess body weight than the body mass index (BMI) since it differentiates between the weight of your fat mass and your body mass. Estimating your percentage body fat can be valuable to monitor your progress during Perfect Weight America.

# Determining Your Perfect Weight

There are many methods for calculating body fat, but the simplest way would be to visit a local fitness club. Even if you're not a member, most club staff would be willing to test you with a handheld electronic body fat analyzer (which costs $50–$75 online) or use skin-fold calipers to pinch several strategic areas of your body, like the triceps, chest, waist, and thigh.

If a fitness club isn't convenient, you can go online and find any number of body fat calculators. Be sure to have a cloth tape measure handy. While different calculators use different formulas, you will often be asked to measure the circumference of your waist, hips, forearm, and wrist. Both HealthCentral.com and drsears.com have excellent tests, or just type in "home body fat test" or "body fat calculator" in the search bar.

## Waist Size

Did you know that the circumference of your waist, not your overall weight, is the leading indicator of mortality related to being overweight? The closer your waist is to "perfect," the healthier you will be. For women, a generally recommended waist size is 32 inches—with dangerous health consequences increasing when 35 inches is reached and exceeded. For men, a generally recommended waist size is 35 inches—with dangerous health consequences increasing when 40 inches is reached and exceeded.

| Risk of Associated Disease According to BMI and Waist Size | | | |
|---|---|---|---|
| BMI | | Waist less than or equal to 40 in. (men) or 35 in. (women) | Waist greater than 40 in. (men) or 35 in. (women) |
| 18.5 or less | Underweight | N/A | N/A |
| 18.5–24.9 | Normal | N/A | N/A |
| 25.0–29.9 | Overweight | Increased | High |
| 30.0–34.9 | Obese | High | Very High |
| 35.0–39.9 | Obese | Very High | Very High |
| 40 or greater | Extremely Obese | Extremely High | Extremely High |

You should now have a strong idea of what your perfect weight should be, although the whole point of these measurements and calculations is that there is no "perfect weight" that can be applied across the board. God created everyone differently, and our bodies change shape as we grow older. By listening to your body and understanding BMI, frame size, body fat, muscle mass, and waist size, you will see steady progress as you strive toward your perfect weight.

You will find a table on page 15 where you can record all of the measurements and calculations discussed in this section, which will help you realize when you've arrived at your perfect weight.

# The Perfect Weight Checklist

The biggest step of all is always the first one. Before embarking on any weight-loss decision and action, build a support team around you. Include your family members, friends, and co-workers as well as your primary care physician. Tell them that you will need their encouragement as well their accountability during this endeavor.

Although the ultimate responsibility for success sits squarely on your shoulders, having a support team will bolster your spirits during the difficult moments ahead. When taking the biggest step, it's a good idea to explore why certain "diets" haven't worked in the past, why you've overeaten, or why you've missed the boat. Taking an honest audit of your life is by no means an easy process, but it is a profitable one in terms of transformation.

Once you've looked inward and asked yourself some tough questions, communicate your intentions to friends and family that it's time to move forward. In a nutshell, here are the commitments we'd love to see you make:

- Commit to detoxing your body with a seasonal Perfect Cleanse regimen before embarking on your sixteen-week Perfect Weight experience. See *Perfect Weight America* for details.

- Commit to following the sixteen-week nutrition and diet program laid out in *Perfect Weight America*.

- Commit to completing a Perfect Weight Health Questionnaire online at www.PerfectWeightAmerica.com.

- Write a description of your current state of health, how you feel about yourself, what you'd like to see changed in sixteen weeks, and what you see yourself becoming during this time. For your convenience, we have provided a place for you to record your goals for Phase I on page 16; Phase II, page 50; Phrase III, page 84; and Phase IV, page 118.

- Determine a goal for where you want your perfect weight to be. Record this goal along with the following measurements on page 15.

- Calculate key measurements (weight, height, BMI, body fat, and waist measurement) so that you have a valid "before" snapshot of your health. Record these measurements on page 15 of this journal.

We also recommend the following health measurements be made for your reference as well as to monitor progress. We've provided a place to document these measurements on page 15 as well.

- Blood pressure
- Resting heart rate
- Full body photo

Have blood work done, including the following tests.*

- Homocysteine
- Lipid Panel
- Serum Albumin
- Complete Blood Count
- Blood Glucose Test/Fasting Glucose Test
- Lipid Peroxide Assessment

Commit to shopping for the right foods. Prepare your grocery list, based on each phase you enter. This may include:

- Cleaning out processed and sugary foods from your pantry

- Choosing healthy and organic grocery items at your local grocery store or health food store

- Purchasing some items through e-tailers and online suppliers

Commit to recording what you eat, the supplements you take, the water you drink, and the exercise you complete, well as journaling your thoughts and experiences in the *Perfect Weight Journal*.

Commit to attending periodic meetings and weigh-ins at a local Perfect Weight America chapter, if applicable. For information on the Perfect Weight America program nearest you, visit our Web site at www.PerfectWeightAmerica.com.

Commit to purchasing the following supplements, which are available at your local health food store or through online e-tailers.

---

* Wellness blood work might be covered by your insurance. Consult with your primary care physician to discuss the result of your blood work before and after you complete the program.

- Four bottles of Living Multi Optimal Formula, 252 count
- Four bottles of Olde World Icelandic Cod Liver Oil, 8 oz.
- Four bottles of fücoTHIN non-stimulant thermogenic, 90 count

Commit to healthy snacking. We recommend the following snacks, which have been designed to nourish, satiate, and control the appetite. These snacks are available at your local health food store or through online e-tailers.

- Perfect Meal (for Phase I through Phase III)
- Perfec Weight America or Garden of Life Organic Food bars (for Phase II through Phase III)
- Garden of Life Rainforest Cacao Chocolate (for Phase III through Phase IV)

Review other educational resources, books, and Web sites that we recommend on page 12 of this journal.

## Phase I (Week 1–Week 4)

This sixteen-week program is laid out in complete detail in the book *Perfect Weight America*. Here is a reminder of what the four phases entail. Phase I, the "purification" stage, is the most rigorous and challenging part of the diet but also the most rewarding. You'll see in the approved foods lists in *Perfect Weight America* that white sugar, artificial sweeteners, and preservatives are *verboten*. Not eating these foods often causes temporary withdrawal-type symptoms such as headaches, carbohydrate cravings, less energy, mood swings, or even changes in your bowel habits. These "detox" reactions are indications that the program is working as the body works to cleanse toxins from the system. When you have the "blahs," increase water intake and rest.

Phase I is designed to stabilize blood sugar levels, reduce inflammation, enhance digestion, and balance hormone levels in the body. This phase restricts disaccharide-heavy carbohydrate foods such as pastas and breads but makes up for it in the variety of delicious, filling foods you can enjoy. You are more likely to see most of your weight loss during this phase due to consuming carbohydrate-restrictive foods. There is also the added benefit of improved digestion, smoother skin, and increased energy levels. For a complete list of foods that are aproved, along with what foods to avoid during Phase I, see pages 118–123 in *Perfect Weight America*.

During Phase I, it is recommended that you do not drink any alcohol—wine, beer, or mixed drinks—but you are allowed two "cheat" meals per week. The best time to cheat is on the weekend, but do not eat any of the foods marked "Avoid" in *Perfect Weight America*. Try to keep your cheating within a sixty-minute period so the body doesn't release more insulin into the bloodstream.

## Phase II (Week 5–Week 8)

Phase II allows for a greater variety of foods, but weight loss is not as rapid during this phase. The most important point of Phase II is to maintain blood sugar levels and create and instill healthy eating habits that can last a lifetime. During Phase II, you're cleared to eat more foods, which are listed on pages 123–125 of *Perfect Weight America*. Remember, you should still not drink any alcohol: wine, beer, or mixed drinks. Keep your cheat meals to a minimum; no more than one or two a week.

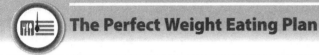

# The Perfect Weight Eating Plan

## Phase III (Week 9–Week 12)

Phase III allows you to increase the varieties of foods as well as more carbohydrates into the diet. You may be wondering, "Can I maintain weight loss by eating carbohydrates again?"

The answer is yes! Carbohydrates do have a place in our diets and bodies, but the carbs must be in their natural and unrefined state. Fuel your body with simple whole fruits and honey, complex sprouted grains, delightful beans, and healthy vegetables. Supplying your body with natural carbohydrates will help you to balance the chemical processes in your body and keep you healthy. A complete list of what you are and are not allowed to eat during Phase III can be found on page 125 in *Perfect Weight America*.

It is still recommended that you not drink any alcohol, but if it's a special occasion, organic red wine is preferred. Organic wines contain some antioxidant benefits when used in moderation. Red wines contain more of these benefits than white wines. We do not recommend the use of any mixed drinks.

## Phase IV (Week 13–Week 16)

Phase IV is the "lifestyle" phase that will allow you to maintain your perfect weight. As you approach your perfect weight, you should notice significant improvements in your health. If you're feeling great and feeling like you've reached your perfect weight, then continue on this lifestyle phase.

Phase IV also provides you the opportunity to step back and ask some questions: Have you reached the goals you set for yourself? Do you feel and look the way you want? If you are still suffering from symptoms related to insulin resistance or you feel like you've gotten off track, then use this time period to implement Phase I or Phase II again.

You're cleared to resume drinking alcohol, but in moderate amounts. Don't forget that alcohol has twice as many calories per gram as protein or carbohydrates. Cheat meals should be a thing of the past, as well as your cravings for junk food.

Eat meals balanced with healthy proteins and fats, watch your portion size, eliminate refined foods, and maintain regular exercise into your week.

# The Perfect Weight Supplement Regimen

Complete information on the following regimen to achieve success on the Perfect Weight America program is provided in *Perfect Weight America*. Here's a summary of the supplements that are recommended. Caution: As with any dietary supplement, consult your health-care practitioner before using this product, especially if you are pregnant, nursing, or under medical supervision.

## Nonstimulant Thermogenic

### fücoTHIN

- Take one to four capsules three times daily with each meal (total of three to ten capsules daily).
- If using an equivalent supplement, follow manufacturer's suggested usage.

## Whole-Food Multivitamin

### Living Multi Men's or Women's Optimal Formula*

- Take two or three tablets three times daily, at each meal (six to nine tablets daily).
- If using an equivalent supplement, follow manufacturer's suggested usage.

## Cod Liver Oil

### Olde World Icelandic Cod Liver Oil**

- Take 1 to 3 teaspoons nightly, right before dinner.
- If using CODmega Wild Fish & Cod Liver Oil Complex, take three to nine capsules nightly, right before dinner.
- If using an equivalent supplement, follow manufacturer's suggested usage.

---

\* Warning: An accidental overdose of iron-containing products is a leading cause of fatal poisoning in children less than six years of age. Keep out of reach of children. In case of accidental overdose, call a physician or poison control center immediately.

\*\* Warning: Do not take this product if you are using blood thinners or anticipate surgery. Consult with a physician before taking this product if you are pregnant, diabetic, or sensitive to iodine. Keep out of the reach of children.

### Web Sites to Check Out

#### www.PerfectWeightAmerica.com

This online resource will be your personal Perfect Weight coach as well as a place that will provide you with a detailed, individualized daily health and wellness plan covering diet, supplementation, exercise, toxin levels, and stress management.

When you fill out a health questionnaire on www.PerfectWeightAmerica.com, you will become part of an online community with access to multiple tools to keep you on track: daily reminders, an online journal, shopping lists, etc. We believe that PerfectWeightAmerica.com will give you a road map that you can follow to experience the type of health and wellness that you haven't known for years or perhaps even decades.

The cost is free for the first twelve months to everyone who's obtained a copy of *Perfect Weight America* or this journal. Type in PWA as your access code.

You can also visit Jordan Rubin's Web site at www.JordanRubin.com, where you can claim your Extraordinary Health Gift Pack. This pack comes with *The Maker's Diet* book, a *Shopping for Optimal Health* DVD, a CD on the benefits of whole-food supplementation, a subscription to Dr. Mercola's e-Healthy e-newsletter, a Garden of Life Organic Super Seed Whole Food Fiber Bar, and a Perfect Meal vanilla packet at no charge. You must visit this Web site to take advantage of these valuable foods and resources integral to the Perfect Weight America plan.

You can also visit www.WeekendOfWellness.com to learn more about special weekend events hosted by Jordan Rubin and his team of doctors and health experts. Held in different cities across the country, these weekend programs are designed to provide knowledge and practical skills and a cutting-edge health education. Whether you are a health professional, personal trainer, health food storeowner, or an individual who is serious about your health, the Weekend of Wellness is for you.

Other recommended Web sites include:

## www.westonaprice.org

The Weston A. Price Foundation is a nonprofit, tax-exempt charity founded in 1999 to disseminate the research of nutrition pioneer Dr. Weston Price, whose studies of isolated non-industrialized peoples established the parameters of human health and determined the optimum characteristics of human diets.

## www.mercola.com

This Web site founded by Dr. Joseph Mercola contains a vast amount of the latest health information and commentary by Dr. Mercola; it reaches hundreds of thousands of people each week.

## www.gardenoflife.com

Garden of Life provides supplements for digestive health, foundational nutrition, immunity support, optimal wellness, and weight management, as well as a line of living foods and personal care products. This Web site not only discusses these products in detail but also educates on topics like the digestive system, sleep and rest, fasting, functional fitness, positive thinking, and more.

### Books

*Nourishing Traditions: The Cookbook That Challenges Politically Correct Nutrition and the Diet Dictocrats* by Sally Fallon and Mary G. Enig, PhD

This well-researched guide to traditional foods dispels the myths of low-fat diets while providing sound nutritional education. Sally Fallon lists practical and delicious recipes in addition to proper preparation of whole-grain products, easy-to-prepare enzyme-enriched condiments and beverages, and appropriate diets for babies and children.

*Nutrition and Physical Degeneration* by Weston A. Price

In the 1930s, Weston A. Price, a dentist and independent nutrition researcher, traveled to various isolated parts of the earth where the inhabitants had no contact with "civilization" to study their health and physical development. The photographs Price took, the descriptions of what he found, and his startling conclusions are preserved in a book considered a masterpiece by many nutrition researchers.

## DVDs

*Functional Fitness*, available from www.JordanRubin.com

*Shopping for Optimal Health*, available from www.JordanRubin.com

# Health Assessment Table

(Consult your physician before beginning this program.)

**Your Perfect Weight\* (pounds):** _____

| Beginning Date: _____ | Before | After Phase I | After Phase II | After Phase III | After Phase IV |
|---|---|---|---|---|---|
| **Anthropometric Measurements** | | | | | |
| Weight (pounds) | | | | | |
| Height (inches) | | | | | |
| Hips\*\* (pounds) | | | | | |
| Waist\*\*\* (inches) | | | | | |
| Wrist\*\* (inches) | | | | | |
| Forearm\*\* (inches) | | | | | |
| Frame size (ratio) | | | | | |
| **Statistical Measurements** | | | | | |
| BMI (kg/m2) | | | | | |
| Body fat (%) | | | | | |
| **Heart Health Measurements** | | | | | |
| Blood pressure, systolic (mmHg) | | | | | |
| Blood pressure, diastolic (mmHg) | | | | | |
| Pulse/resting heart rate (bpm) | | | | | |
| **Blood work (write in tests and results)** | | | | | |
| | | | | | |
| | | | | | |
| | | | | | |
| | | | | | |
| | | | | | |
| | | | | | |
| | | | | | |
| | | | | | |
| | | | | | |

\* You know your body. Use your perception and the data in this chart to set a goal for your perfect weight.

\*\* Measure at widest point.

\*\*\* Measure at navel.

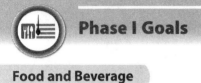

## Phase I Goals

### Food and Beverage

I will add the following foods to my eating (see pages 118–123 of *Perfect Weight America* for a complete list of allowed foods):

_____

_____

_____

I will avoid eating the following foods (see pages 118–123 of *Perfect Weight America* for a complete list of foods to avoid):

_____

_____

_____

I will drink _____ ounces of water daily.

I will avoid drinking the following beverages:

_____

_____

_____

I will add the following healthy snacks to my daily snacking regimen:

_____

_____

_____

I will avoid the following snack foods:

_____

_____

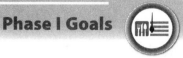

## Supplements

I will take the following supplements daily:

_____

_____

## Exercise and Fitness Goals

I will do the following exercises at least four to five times a week:

_____

_____

_____

## Rest

I will go to bed by _____ each night.

## Other Goals for Phase I

_____

_____

_____

_____

_____

_____

_____

_____

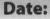

### Record everything you consume, including food, snacks, supplements, water, mints, and gum.

**Breakfast**

Water:
Supplements:
Morning snack:

**Lunch**

Water:
Supplements:
Midday snack:

**Dinner**

Water:
Supplements:
Evening snack:

**Exercise**

**HEALING CODES: Do the Healing Codes exercise on page 189 in *Perfect Weight America*. Record your stress level as you rated it while doing the exercise.**

| Healing Codes (AM) | Beginning: | End: | 10 min. later: |
| Healing Codes (PM) | Beginning: | End: | 10 min. later: |

Did you meet your Phase I goals today? _____

Record your thoughts, insights, and questions; your emotional outlook and physical state; and your successes and challenges.

_____

_____

_____

| **Record everything you consume, including food, snacks, supplements, water, mints, and gum.** |
|---|

**Breakfast**
_____

_____

_____

Water: _____
Supplements: _____
Morning snack: _____

**Lunch**
_____

_____

_____

Water: _____
Supplements: _____
Midday snack: _____

**Dinner**
_____

_____

_____

Water: _____
Supplements: _____
Evening snack: _____

**Exercise**
_____

_____

| **HEALING CODES: Do the Healing Codes exercise on page 189 in *Perfect Weight America*. Record your stress level as you rated it while doing the exercise.** | | | |
|---|---|---|---|
| Healing Codes (AM) | Beginning: | End: | 10 min. later: |
| Healing Codes (PM) | Beginning: | End: | 10 min. later: |

Did you meet your Phase I goals today? _____

Record your thoughts, insights, and questions; your emotional outlook and physical state; and your successes and challenges.

_____

_____

_____

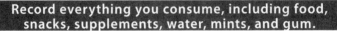

## Phase I, Week 1, Day 3        Date: _____

**Record everything you consume, including food, snacks, supplements, water, mints, and gum.**

**Breakfast**

Water:
Supplements:
Morning snack:

**Lunch**

Water:
Supplements:
Midday snack:

**Dinner**

Water:
Supplements:
Evening snack:

**Exercise**

**HEALING CODES: Do the Healing Codes exercise on page 189 in *Perfect Weight America*. Record your stress level as you rated it while doing the exercise.**

| Healing Codes (AM) | Beginning: | End: | 10 min. later: |
| Healing Codes (PM) | Beginning: | End: | 10 min. later: |

Did you meet your Phase I goals today? _____

Record your thoughts, insights, and questions; your emotional outlook and physical state; and your successes and challenges.

_____

_____

_____

## Record everything you consume, including food, snacks, supplements, water, mints, and gum.

**Breakfast**

Water:

Supplements:

Morning snack:

**Lunch**

Water:

Supplements:

Midday snack:

**Dinner**

Water:

Supplements:

Evening snack:

**Exercise**

**HEALING CODES:** Do the Healing Codes exercise on page 189 in *Perfect Weight America*. Record your stress level as you rated it while doing the exercise.

| Healing Codes (AM) | Beginning: | End: | 10 min. later: |
| Healing Codes (PM) | Beginning: | End: | 10 min. later: |

Did you meet your Phase I goals today? _____

Record your thoughts, insights, and questions; your emotional outlook and physical state; and your successes and challenges.

**Record everything you consume, including food, snacks, supplements, water, mints, and gum.**

**Breakfast**

Water:
Supplements:
Morning snack:

**Lunch**

Water:
Supplements:
Midday snack:

**Dinner**

Water:
Supplements:
Evening snack:

**Exercise**

**HEALING CODES: Do the Healing Codes exercise on page 189 in *Perfect Weight America*. Record your stress level as you rated it while doing the exercise.**

| Healing Codes (AM) | Beginning: | End: | 10 min. later: |
| Healing Codes (PM) | Beginning: | End: | 10 min. later: |

Did you meet your Phase I goals today? _____

Record your thoughts, insights, and questions; your emotional outlook and physical state; and your successes and challenges.

_____

_____

_____

**Record everything you consume, including food, snacks, supplements, water, mints, and gum.**

**Breakfast**

Water:

Supplements:

Morning snack:

**Lunch**

Water:

Supplements:

Midday snack:

**Dinner**

Water:

Supplements:

Evening snack:

**Exercise**

**HEALING CODES: Do the Healing Codes exercise on page 189 in *Perfect Weight America*. Record your stress level as you rated it while doing the exercise.**

| Healing Codes (AM) | Beginning: | End: | 10 min. later: |
| Healing Codes (PM) | Beginning: | End: | 10 min. later: |

Did you meet your Phase I goals today? _____

Record your thoughts, insights, and questions; your emotional outlook and physical state; and your successes and challenges.

_____

_____

_____

**Record everything you consume, including food, snacks, supplements, water, mints, and gum.**

**Breakfast**

Water:

Supplements:

Morning snack:

**Lunch**

Water:

Supplements:

Midday snack:

**Dinner**

Water:

Supplements:

Evening snack:

**Exercise**

**HEALING CODES: Do the Healing Codes exercise on page 189 in *Perfect Weight America*. Record your stress level as you rated it while doing the exercise.**

| Healing Codes (AM) | Beginning: | End: | 10 min. later: |
|---|---|---|---|
| Healing Codes (PM) | Beginning: | End: | 10 min. later: |

Did you meet your Phase I goals today? _____

Record your thoughts, insights, and questions; your emotional outlook and physical state; and your successes and challenges.

_____

_____

_____

# Summary of Week 1

How many days did you follow the Perfect Weight Eating Plan? _____

How many days did you take the recommended supplements? _____

How many days did you drink at least half your body weight in ounces of water?

_____

How many days did you meet your goals for Phase I? _____

How many days did you exercise this week? _____

Write down any extra thoughts you want to capture about your week.

_____

_____

_____

_____

_____

_____

_____

_____

_____

_____

_____

_____

_____

_____

_____

_____

_____

**Record everything you consume, including food, snacks, supplements, water, mints, and gum.**

Breakfast

Water:
Supplements:
Morning snack:

Lunch

Water:
Supplements:
Midday snack:

Dinner

Water:
Supplements:
Evening snack:

Exercise

**HEALING CODES: Do the Healing Codes exercise on page 189 in *Perfect Weight America*. Record your stress level as you rated it while doing the exercise.**

| Healing Codes (AM) | Beginning: | End: | 10 min. later: |
| Healing Codes (PM) | Beginning: | End: | 10 min. later: |

Did you meet your Phase I goals today? _____

Record your thoughts, insights, and questions; your emotional outlook and physical state; and your successes and challenges.

_____

_____

_____

| Record everything you consume, including food, snacks, supplements, water, mints, and gum. |
| :-- |

**Breakfast**


Water:
Supplements:
Morning snack:

**Lunch**


Water:
Supplements:
Midday snack:

**Dinner**


Water:
Supplements:
Evening snack:

**Exercise**


**HEALING CODES:** Do the Healing Codes exercise on page 189 in *Perfect Weight America*. Record your stress level as you rated it while doing the exercise.

| Healing Codes (AM) | Beginning: | End: | 10 min. later: |
| --- | --- | --- | --- |
| Healing Codes (PM) | Beginning: | End: | 10 min. later: |

Did you meet your Phase I goals today? _____

Record your thoughts, insights, and questions; your emotional outlook and physical state; and your successes and challenges.

_____

_____

_____

**Record everything you consume, including food, snacks, supplements, water, mints, and gum.**

Breakfast

Water:
Supplements:
Morning snack:

Lunch

Water:
Supplements:
Midday snack:

Dinner

Water:
Supplements:
Evening snack:

Exercise

**HEALING CODES: Do the Healing Codes exercise on page 189 in *Perfect Weight America*. Record your stress level as you rated it while doing the exercise.**

| Healing Codes (AM) | Beginning: | End: | 10 min. later: |
| Healing Codes (PM) | Beginning: | End: | 10 min. later: |

Did you meet your Phase I goals today? _____

Record your thoughts, insights, and questions; your emotional outlook and physical state; and your successes and challenges.

_____

_____

_____

| Record everything you consume, including food, snacks, supplements, water, mints, and gum. |
|---|

**Breakfast**

|  |
|---|
|  |
|  |
| Water: |
| Supplements: |
| Morning snack: |

**Lunch**

|  |
|---|
|  |
|  |
| Water: |
| Supplements: |
| Midday snack: |

**Dinner**

|  |
|---|
|  |
|  |
| Water: |
| Supplements: |
| Evening snack: |

**Exercise**

|  |
|---|

| HEALING CODES: Do the Healing Codes exercise on page 189 in *Perfect Weight America*. Record your stress level as you rated it while doing the exercise. | | | |
|---|---|---|---|
| Healing Codes (AM) | Beginning: | End: | 10 min. later: |
| Healing Codes (PM) | Beginning: | End: | 10 min. later: |

Did you meet your Phase I goals today? _____

Record your thoughts, insights, and questions; your emotional outlook and physical state; and your successes and challenges.

_____

_____

_____

## Record everything you consume, including food, snacks, supplements, water, mints, and gum.

**Breakfast**

Water:
Supplements:
Morning snack:

**Lunch**

Water:
Supplements:
Midday snack:

**Dinner**

Water:
Supplements:
Evening snack:

**Exercise**

**HEALING CODES: Do the Healing Codes exercise on page 189 in *Perfect Weight America*. Record your stress level as you rated it while doing the exercise.**

| Healing Codes (AM) | Beginning: | End: | 10 min. later: |
| Healing Codes (PM) | Beginning: | End: | 10 min. later: |

Did you meet your Phase I goals today? _____

Record your thoughts, insights, and questions; your emotional outlook and physical state; and your successes and challenges.

_____

_____

_____

| Record everything you consume, including food, snacks, supplements, water, mints, and gum. |
| --- |

**Breakfast**



Water:
Supplements:
Morning snack:

**Lunch**



Water:
Supplements:
Midday snack:

**Dinner**



Water:
Supplements:
Evening snack:

**Exercise**


**HEALING CODES:** Do the Healing Codes exercise on page 189 in *Perfect Weight America*. Record your stress level as you rated it while doing the exercise.

| Healing Codes (AM) | Beginning: | End: | 10 min. later: |
| --- | --- | --- | --- |
| Healing Codes (PM) | Beginning: | End: | 10 min. later: |

Did you meet your Phase I goals today? _____

Record your thoughts, insights, and questions; your emotional outlook and physical state; and your successes and challenges.

_____

_____

_____

## Record everything you consume, including food, snacks, supplements, water, mints, and gum.

**Breakfast**



Water:
Supplements:
Morning snack:

**Lunch**



Water:
Supplements:
Midday snack:

**Dinner**



Water:
Supplements:
Evening snack:

**Exercise**


**HEALING CODES: Do the Healing Codes exercise on page 189 in *Perfect Weight America*. Record your stress level as you rated it while doing the exercise.**

| Healing Codes (AM) | Beginning: | End: | 10 min. later: |
| Healing Codes (PM) | Beginning: | End: | 10 min. later: |

Did you meet your Phase I goals today? _____

Record your thoughts, insights, and questions; your emotional outlook and physical state; and your successes and challenges.

_____

_____

_____

## Summary of Week 2

How many days did you follow the Perfect Weight Eating Plan? _____

How many days did you take the recommended supplements? _____

How many days did you drink at least half your body weight in ounces of water?

_____

How many days did you meet your goals for Phase I? _____

How many days did you exercise this week? _____

Write down any extra thoughts you want to capture about your week.

_____

_____

_____

_____

_____

_____

_____

_____

_____

_____

_____

_____

_____

_____

**Record everything you consume, including food, snacks, supplements, water, mints, and gum.**

**Breakfast**

Water:
Supplements:
Morning snack:

**Lunch**

Water:
Supplements:
Midday snack:

**Dinner**

Water:
Supplements:
Evening snack:

**Exercise**

**HEALING CODES: Do the Healing Codes exercise on page 189 in *Perfect Weight America*. Record your stress level as you rated it while doing the exercise.**

| Healing Codes (AM) | Beginning: | End: | 10 min. later: |
| Healing Codes (PM) | Beginning: | End: | 10 min. later: |

Did you meet your Phase I goals today? _____

Record your thoughts, insights, and questions; your emotional outlook and physical state; and your successes and challenges.

_____

_____

_____

## Record everything you consume, including food, snacks, supplements, water, mints, and gum.

**Breakfast**

Water:

Supplements:

Morning snack:

**Lunch**

Water:

Supplements:

Midday snack:

**Dinner**

Water:

Supplements:

Evening snack:

**Exercise**

---

**HEALING CODES: Do the Healing Codes exercise on page 189 in *Perfect Weight America*. Record your stress level as you rated it while doing the exercise.**

| Healing Codes (AM) | Beginning: | End: | 10 min. later: |
|---|---|---|---|
| Healing Codes (PM) | Beginning: | End: | 10 min. later: |

Did you meet your Phase I goals today? _____

Record your thoughts, insights, and questions; your emotional outlook and physical state; and your successes and challenges.

_____

_____

_____

**Record everything you consume, including food, snacks, supplements, water, mints, and gum.**

**Breakfast**

Water:

Supplements:

Morning snack:

**Lunch**

Water:

Supplements:

Midday snack:

**Dinner**

Water:

Supplements:

Evening snack:

**Exercise**

**HEALING CODES: Do the Healing Codes exercise on page 189 in *Perfect Weight America*. Record your stress level as you rated it while doing the exercise.**

| Healing Codes (AM) | Beginning: | End: | 10 min. later: |
| Healing Codes (PM) | Beginning: | End: | 10 min. later: |

Did you meet your Phase I goals today? _____

Record your thoughts, insights, and questions; your emotional outlook and physical state; and your successes and challenges.

_____

_____

_____

| Record everything you consume, including food, snacks, supplements, water, mints, and gum. |
|---|

**Breakfast**

Water:
Supplements:
Morning snack:

**Lunch**

Water:
Supplements:
Midday snack:

**Dinner**

Water:
Supplements:
Evening snack:

**Exercise**

**HEALING CODES:** Do the Healing Codes exercise on page 189 in *Perfect Weight America*. Record your stress level as you rated it while doing the exercise.

| Healing Codes (AM) | Beginning: | End: | 10 min. later: |
|---|---|---|---|
| Healing Codes (PM) | Beginning: | End: | 10 min. later: |

Did you meet your Phase I goals today? _____

Record your thoughts, insights, and questions; your emotional outlook and physical state; and your successes and challenges.

_____

_____

_____

**Record everything you consume, including food, snacks, supplements, water, mints, and gum.**

**Breakfast**

Water:
Supplements:
Morning snack:

**Lunch**

Water:
Supplements:
Midday snack:

**Dinner**

Water:
Supplements:
Evening snack:

**Exercise**

**HEALING CODES: Do the Healing Codes exercise on page 189 in *Perfect Weight America*. Record your stress level as you rated it while doing the exercise.**

| Healing Codes (AM) | Beginning: | End: | 10 min. later: |
| Healing Codes (PM) | Beginning: | End: | 10 min. later: |

Did you meet your Phase I goals today? _____

Record your thoughts, insights, and questions; your emotional outlook and physical state; and your successes and challenges.

_____

_____

_____

**Record everything you consume, including food, snacks, supplements, water, mints, and gum.**

**Breakfast**

Water:
Supplements:
Morning snack:

**Lunch**

Water:
Supplements:
Midday snack:

**Dinner**

Water:
Supplements:
Evening snack:

**Exercise**

**HEALING CODES: Do the Healing Codes exercise on page 189 in *Perfect Weight America*. Record your stress level as you rated it while doing the exercise.**

| Healing Codes (AM) | Beginning: | End: | 10 min. later: |
| Healing Codes (PM) | Beginning: | End: | 10 min. later: |

Did you meet your Phase I goals today? _____

Record your thoughts, insights, and questions; your emotional outlook and physical state; and your successes and challenges.

_____

_____

_____

**Record everything you consume, including food, snacks, supplements, water, mints, and gum.**

**Breakfast**

Water:
Supplements:
Morning snack:

**Lunch**

Water:
Supplements:
Midday snack:

**Dinner**

Water:
Supplements:
Evening snack:

**Exercise**

**HEALING CODES: Do the Healing Codes exercise on page 189 in *Perfect Weight America*. Record your stress level as you rated it while doing the exercise.**

| Healing Codes (AM) | Beginning: | End: | 10 min. later: |
| Healing Codes (PM) | Beginning: | End: | 10 min. later: |

Did you meet your Phase I goals today? _____

Record your thoughts, insights, and questions; your emotional outlook and physical state; and your successes and challenges.

_____

_____

_____

# Summary of Week 3

How many days did you follow the Perfect Weight Eating Plan? _____

How many days did you take the recommended supplements? _____

How many days did you drink at least half your body weight in ounces of water?

_____

How many days did you meet your goals for Phase I? _____

How many days did you exercise this week? _____

Write down any extra thoughts you want to capture about your week.

_____

_____

_____

_____

_____

_____

_____

_____

_____

_____

_____

_____

_____

_____

_____

**Record everything you consume, including food, snacks, supplements, water, mints, and gum.**

Breakfast

Water:
Supplements:
Morning snack:

Lunch

Water:
Supplements:
Midday snack:

Dinner

Water:
Supplements:
Evening snack:

Exercise

**HEALING CODES: Do the Healing Codes exercise on page 189 in *Perfect Weight America*. Record your stress level as you rated it while doing the exercise.**

| Healing Codes (AM) | Beginning: | End: | 10 min. later: |
| Healing Codes (PM) | Beginning: | End: | 10 min. later: |

Did you meet your Phase I goals today? _____

Record your thoughts, insights, and questions; your emotional outlook and physical state; and your successes and challenges.

_____

_____

_____

| Record everything you consume, including food, snacks, supplements, water, mints, and gum. |
|---|

**Breakfast**

Water:
Supplements:
Morning snack:

**Lunch**

Water:
Supplements:
Midday snack:

**Dinner**

Water:
Supplements:
Evening snack:

**Exercise**

**HEALING CODES:** Do the Healing Codes exercise on page 189 in *Perfect Weight America*. Record your stress level as you rated it while doing the exercise.

| Healing Codes (AM) | Beginning: | End: | 10 min. later: |
|---|---|---|---|
| Healing Codes (PM) | Beginning: | End: | 10 min. later: |

Did you meet your Phase I goals today? _____

Record your thoughts, insights, and questions; your emotional outlook and physical state; and your successes and challenges.

_____

_____

_____

**Record everything you consume, including food, snacks, supplements, water, mints, and gum.**

Breakfast

Water:
Supplements:
Morning snack:

Lunch

Water:
Supplements:
Midday snack:

Dinner

Water:
Supplements:
Evening snack:

Exercise

**HEALING CODES: Do the Healing Codes exercise on page 189 in *Perfect Weight America*. Record your stress level as you rated it while doing the exercise.**

| Healing Codes (AM) | Beginning: | End: | 10 min. later: |
| Healing Codes (PM) | Beginning: | End: | 10 min. later: |

Did you meet your Phase I goals today? _____

Record your thoughts, insights, and questions; your emotional outlook and physical state; and your successes and challenges.

_____

_____

_____

| Record everything you consume, including food, snacks, supplements, water, mints, and gum. |
|---|

**Breakfast**




Water:
Supplements:
Morning snack:

**Lunch**




Water:
Supplements:
Midday snack:

**Dinner**




Water:
Supplements:
Evening snack:

**Exercise**


**HEALING CODES:** Do the Healing Codes exercise on page 189 in *Perfect Weight America*. Record your stress level as you rated it while doing the exercise.

| Healing Codes (AM) | Beginning: | End: | 10 min. later: |
|---|---|---|---|
| Healing Codes (PM) | Beginning: | End: | 10 min. later: |

Did you meet your Phase I goals today? _____

Record your thoughts, insights, and questions; your emotional outlook and physical state; and your successes and challenges.

_____

_____

_____

### Record everything you consume, including food, snacks, supplements, water, mints, and gum.

**Breakfast**

Water:
Supplements:
Morning snack:

**Lunch**

Water:
Supplements:
Midday snack:

**Dinner**

Water:
Supplements:
Evening snack:

**Exercise**

### HEALING CODES: Do the Healing Codes exercise on page 189 in *Perfect Weight America*. Record your stress level as you rated it while doing the exercise.

| Healing Codes (AM) | Beginning: | End: | 10 min. later: |
| Healing Codes (PM) | Beginning: | End: | 10 min. later: |

Did you meet your Phase I goals today? _____

Record your thoughts, insights, and questions; your emotional outlook and physical state; and your successes and challenges.

_____

_____

_____

**Record everything you consume, including food, snacks, supplements, water, mints, and gum.**

**Breakfast**

Water:
Supplements:
Morning snack:

**Lunch**

Water:
Supplements:
Midday snack:

**Dinner**

Water:
Supplements:
Evening snack:

**Exercise**

**HEALING CODES: Do the Healing Codes exercise on page 189 in *Perfect Weight America*. Record your stress level as you rated it while doing the exercise.**

| Healing Codes (AM) | Beginning: | End: | 10 min. later: |
| Healing Codes (PM) | Beginning: | End: | 10 min. later: |

Did you meet your Phase I goals today? _____

Record your thoughts, insights, and questions; your emotional outlook and physical state; and your successes and challenges.

_____

_____

_____

**Record everything you consume, including food, snacks, supplements, water, mints, and gum.**

**Breakfast**

Water:
Supplements:
Morning snack:

**Lunch**

Water:
Supplements:
Midday snack:

**Dinner**

Water:
Supplements:
Evening snack:

**Exercise**

**HEALING CODES:** Do the Healing Codes exercise on page 189 in *Perfect Weight America*. Record your stress level as you rated it while doing the exercise.

| Healing Codes (AM) | Beginning: | End: | 10 min. later: |
| Healing Codes (PM) | Beginning: | End: | 10 min. later: |

Did you meet your Phase I goals today? _____

Record your thoughts, insights, and questions; your emotional outlook and physical state; and your successes and challenges.

_____

_____

_____

## Summary of Week 4

How many days did you follow the Perfect Weight Eating Plan? _____

How many days did you take the recommended supplements? _____

How many days did you drink at least half your body weight in ounces of water?

_____

How many days did you meet your goals for Phase I? _____

How many days did you exercise this week? _____

Write down any extra thoughts you want to capture about your week.

_____

_____

_____

_____

_____

_____

_____

_____

_____

_____

_____

_____

_____

_____

_____

_____

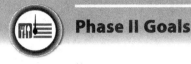

## Phase II Goals

I will continue the progress I made in Phase I.

### Food and Beverage

I will add the following foods to my eating (see pages 123–125 of *Perfect Weight America* for a complete list of allowed foods):

_____

_____

_____

I will avoid eating the following foods (see pages 123–125 of *Perfect Weight America* for a complete list of foods to avoid):

_____

_____

_____

I will drink _____ ounces of water daily.

I will avoid drinking the following beverages:

_____

_____

_____

I will add the following healthy snacks to my daily snacking regimen:

_____

_____

_____

_____

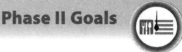

I will avoid the following snack foods:

_____

_____

## Supplements

I will take the following supplements daily:

_____

_____

## Exercise and Fitness Goals

I will do the following exercises at least four to five times a week:

_____

_____

_____

## Rest

I will go to bed by _____ each night.

## Other Goals for Phase II

_____

_____

_____

_____

_____

_____

### Record everything you consume, including food, snacks, supplements, water, mints, and gum.

**Breakfast**

Water:
Supplements:
Morning snack:

**Lunch**

Water:
Supplements:
Midday snack:

**Dinner**

Water:
Supplements:
Evening snack:

**Exercise**

**HEALING CODES: Do the Healing Codes exercise on page 189 in *Perfect Weight America*. Record your stress level as you rated it while doing the exercise.**

| Healing Codes (AM) | Beginning: | End: | 10 min. later: |
| Healing Codes (PM) | Beginning: | End: | 10 min. later: |

Did you meet your Phase II goals today? _____

Record your thoughts, insights, and questions; your emotional outlook and physical state; and your successes and challenges.

_____

_____

_____

| Record everything you consume, including food, snacks, supplements, water, mints, and gum. |
|---|

**Breakfast**




Water:
Supplements:
Morning snack:

**Lunch**




Water:
Supplements:
Midday snack:

**Dinner**




Water:
Supplements:
Evening snack:

**Exercise**


| HEALING CODES: Do the Healing Codes exercise on page 189 in *Perfect Weight America*. Record your stress level as you rated it while doing the exercise. | | | |
|---|---|---|---|
| Healing Codes (AM) | Beginning: | End: | 10 min. later: |
| Healing Codes (PM) | Beginning: | End: | 10 min. later: |

Did you meet your Phase II goals today? _____

Record your thoughts, insights, and questions; your emotional outlook and physical state; and your successes and challenges.

_____

_____

_____

## Record everything you consume, including food, snacks, supplements, water, mints, and gum.

**Breakfast**

Water:
Supplements:
Morning snack:

**Lunch**

Water:
Supplements:
Midday snack:

**Dinner**

Water:
Supplements:
Evening snack:

**Exercise**

**HEALING CODES: Do the Healing Codes exercise on page 189 in *Perfect Weight America*. Record your stress level as you rated it while doing the exercise.**

| Healing Codes (AM) | Beginning: | End: | 10 min. later: |
| Healing Codes (PM) | Beginning: | End: | 10 min. later: |

Did you meet your Phase II goals today? _____

Record your thoughts, insights, and questions; your emotional outlook and physical state; and your successes and challenges.

_____

_____

_____

| Record everything you consume, including food, snacks, supplements, water, mints, and gum. |
| --- |

**Breakfast**



Water:
Supplements:
Morning snack:

**Lunch**



Water:
Supplements:
Midday snack:

**Dinner**



Water:
Supplements:
Evening snack:

**Exercise**


**HEALING CODES: Do the Healing Codes exercise on page 189 in *Perfect Weight America*. Record your stress level as you rated it while doing the exercise.**

| Healing Codes (AM) | Beginning: | End: | 10 min. later: |
| --- | --- | --- | --- |
| Healing Codes (PM) | Beginning: | End: | 10 min. later: |

Did you meet your Phase II goals today? _____

Record your thoughts, insights, and questions; your emotional outlook and physical state; and your successes and challenges.

_____

_____

_____

## Phase II, Week 5, Day 33          Date: _____

**Record everything you consume, including food, snacks, supplements, water, mints, and gum.**

**Breakfast**

Water:
Supplements:
Morning snack:

**Lunch**

Water:
Supplements:
Midday snack:

**Dinner**

Water:
Supplements:
Evening snack:

**Exercise**

**HEALING CODES:** Do the Healing Codes exercise on page 189 in *Perfect Weight America*. Record your stress level as you rated it while doing the exercise.

| Healing Codes (AM) | Beginning: | End: | 10 min. later: |
| Healing Codes (PM) | Beginning: | End: | 10 min. later: |

Did you meet your Phase II goals today? _____

Record your thoughts, insights, and questions; your emotional outlook and physical state; and your successes and challenges.

_____

_____

_____

| Record everything you consume, including food, snacks, supplements, water, mints, and gum. |
|---|

**Breakfast**




Water:
Supplements:
Morning snack:

**Lunch**




Water:
Supplements:
Midday snack:

**Dinner**




Water:
Supplements:
Evening snack:

**Exercise**



**HEALING CODES:** Do the Healing Codes exercise on page 189 in *Perfect Weight America*. Record your stress level as you rated it while doing the exercise.

| Healing Codes (AM) | Beginning: | End: | 10 min. later: |
|---|---|---|---|
| Healing Codes (PM) | Beginning: | End: | 10 min. later: |

Did you meet your Phase II goals today? _____

Record your thoughts, insights, and questions; your emotional outlook and physical state; and your successes and challenges.

_____

_____

_____

### Record everything you consume, including food, snacks, supplements, water, mints, and gum.

**Breakfast**



Water:
Supplements:
Morning snack:

**Lunch**



Water:
Supplements:
Midday snack:

**Dinner**



Water:
Supplements:
Evening snack:

**Exercise**


**HEALING CODES:** Do the Healing Codes exercise on page 189 in *Perfect Weight America*. Record your stress level as you rated it while doing the exercise.

| Healing Codes (AM) | Beginning: | End: | 10 min. later: |
| Healing Codes (PM) | Beginning: | End: | 10 min. later: |

Did you meet your Phase II goals today? _____

Record your thoughts, insights, and questions; your emotional outlook and physical state; and your successes and challenges.

_____

_____

_____

## Summary of Week 5

How many days did you follow the Perfect Weight Eating Plan? _____

How many days did you take the recommended supplements? _____

How many days did you drink at least half your body weight in ounces of water?

_____

How many days did you meet your goals for Phase II? _____

How many days did you exercise this week? _____

Write down any extra thoughts you want to capture about your week.

_____

_____

_____

_____

_____

_____

_____

_____

_____

_____

_____

_____

_____

_____

## Phase II, Week 6, Day 36          Date: _____

### Record everything you consume, including food, snacks, supplements, water, mints, and gum.

**Breakfast**

Water:
Supplements:
Morning snack:

**Lunch**

Water:
Supplements:
Midday snack:

**Dinner**

Water:
Supplements:
Evening snack:

**Exercise**

**HEALING CODES:** Do the Healing Codes exercise on page 189 in *Perfect Weight America*. Record your stress level as you rated it while doing the exercise.

| Healing Codes (AM) | Beginning: | End: | 10 min. later: |
| Healing Codes (PM) | Beginning: | End: | 10 min. later: |

Did you meet your Phase II goals today? _____

Record your thoughts, insights, and questions; your emotional outlook and physical state; and your successes and challenges.

_____

_____

_____

| Record everything you consume, including food, snacks, supplements, water, mints, and gum. |
|---|

**Breakfast**

Water:
Supplements:
Morning snack:

**Lunch**

Water:
Supplements:
Midday snack:

**Dinner**

Water:
Supplements:
Evening snack:

**Exercise**

**HEALING CODES:** Do the Healing Codes exercise on page 189 in *Perfect Weight America*. Record your stress level as you rated it while doing the exercise.

| Healing Codes (AM) | Beginning: | End: | 10 min. later: |
|---|---|---|---|
| Healing Codes (PM) | Beginning: | End: | 10 min. later: |

Did you meet your Phase II goals today? _____

Record your thoughts, insights, and questions; your emotional outlook and physical state; and your successes and challenges.

_____

_____

_____

**Record everything you consume, including food, snacks, supplements, water, mints, and gum.**

**Breakfast**

Water:

Supplements:

Morning snack:

**Lunch**

Water:

Supplements:

Midday snack:

**Dinner**

Water:

Supplements:

Evening snack:

**Exercise**

**HEALING CODES:** Do the Healing Codes exercise on page 189 in *Perfect Weight America*. Record your stress level as you rated it while doing the exercise.

| Healing Codes (AM) | Beginning: | End: | 10 min. later: |
| Healing Codes (PM) | Beginning: | End: | 10 min. later: |

Did you meet your Phase II goals today? _____

Record your thoughts, insights, and questions; your emotional outlook and physical state; and your successes and challenges.

_____

_____

_____

**Date:** _____

| Record everything you consume, including food, snacks, supplements, water, mints, and gum. |
|---|
| **Breakfast** |
| |
| |
| |
| Water: |
| Supplements: |
| Morning snack: |
| **Lunch** |
| |
| |
| |
| Water: |
| Supplements: |
| Midday snack: |
| **Dinner** |
| |
| |
| |
| Water: |
| Supplements: |
| Evening snack: |
| **Exercise** |
| |

| HEALING CODES: Do the Healing Codes exercise on page 189 in *Perfect Weight America*. Record your stress level as you rated it while doing the exercise. | | | |
|---|---|---|---|
| Healing Codes (AM) | Beginning: | End: | 10 min. later: |
| Healing Codes (PM) | Beginning: | End: | 10 min. later: |

Did you meet your Phase II goals today? _____

Record your thoughts, insights, and questions; your emotional outlook and physical state; and your successes and challenges.

_____

_____

_____

**Record everything you consume, including food, snacks, supplements, water, mints, and gum.**

**Breakfast**

Water:
Supplements:
Morning snack:

**Lunch**

Water:
Supplements:
Midday snack:

**Dinner**

Water:
Supplements:
Evening snack:

**Exercise**

**HEALING CODES: Do the Healing Codes exercise on page 189 in *Perfect Weight America*. Record your stress level as you rated it while doing the exercise.**

| Healing Codes (AM) | Beginning: | End: | 10 min. later: |
| Healing Codes (PM) | Beginning: | End: | 10 min. later: |

Did you meet your Phase II goals today? _____

Record your thoughts, insights, and questions; your emotional outlook and physical state; and your successes and challenges.

_____

_____

_____

| Record everything you consume, including food, snacks, supplements, water, mints, and gum. |
|---|
| **Breakfast** |
| |
| |
| |
| Water: |
| Supplements: |
| Morning snack: |
| **Lunch** |
| |
| |
| |
| Water: |
| Supplements: |
| Midday snack: |
| **Dinner** |
| |
| |
| |
| Water: |
| Supplements: |
| Evening snack: |
| **Exercise** |
| |

| HEALING CODES: Do the Healing Codes exercise on page 189 in *Perfect Weight America*. Record your stress level as you rated it while doing the exercise. | | | |
|---|---|---|---|
| Healing Codes (AM) | Beginning: | End: | 10 min. later: |
| Healing Codes (PM) | Beginning: | End: | 10 min. later: |

Did you meet your Phase II goals today? _____

Record your thoughts, insights, and questions; your emotional outlook and physical state; and your successes and challenges.

_____

_____

_____

### Record everything you consume, including food, snacks, supplements, water, mints, and gum.

**Breakfast**

Water:
Supplements:
Morning snack:

**Lunch**

Water:
Supplements:
Midday snack:

**Dinner**

Water:
Supplements:
Evening snack:

**Exercise**

**HEALING CODES:** Do the Healing Codes exercise on page 189 in *Perfect Weight America*. Record your stress level as you rated it while doing the exercise.

| Healing Codes (AM) | Beginning: | End: | 10 min. later: |
|---|---|---|---|
| Healing Codes (PM) | Beginning: | End: | 10 min. later: |

Did you meet your Phase II goals today? _____

Record your thoughts, insights, and questions; your emotional outlook and physical state; and your successes and challenges.

_____

_____

_____

## Summary of Week 6

How many days did you follow the Perfect Weight Eating Plan? _____

How many days did you take the recommended supplements? _____

How many days did you drink at least half your body weight in ounces of water?

_____

How many days did you meet your goals for Phase II? _____

How many days did you exercise this week? _____

Write down any extra thoughts you want to capture about your week.

_____

_____

_____

_____

_____

_____

_____

_____

_____

_____

_____

_____

_____

_____

_____

_____

_____

**Record everything you consume, including food, snacks, supplements, water, mints, and gum.**

**Breakfast**

Water:

Supplements:

Morning snack:

**Lunch**

Water:

Supplements:

Midday snack:

**Dinner**

Water:

Supplements:

Evening snack:

**Exercise**

**HEALING CODES:** Do the Healing Codes exercise on page 189 in *Perfect Weight America*. Record your stress level as you rated it while doing the exercise.

| Healing Codes (AM) | Beginning: | End: | 10 min. later: |
|---|---|---|---|
| Healing Codes (PM) | Beginning: | End: | 10 min. later: |

Did you meet your Phase II goals today? _____

Record your thoughts, insights, and questions; your emotional outlook and physical state; and your successes and challenges.

_____

_____

_____

| Record everything you consume, including food, snacks, supplements, water, mints, and gum. |
|---|

**Breakfast**

Water:
Supplements:
Morning snack:

**Lunch**

Water:
Supplements:
Midday snack:

**Dinner**

Water:
Supplements:
Evening snack:

**Exercise**

**HEALING CODES:** Do the Healing Codes exercise on page 189 in *Perfect Weight America*. Record your stress level as you rated it while doing the exercise.

| Healing Codes (AM) | Beginning: | End: | 10 min. later: |
|---|---|---|---|
| Healing Codes (PM) | Beginning: | End: | 10 min. later: |

Did you meet your Phase II goals today? _____

Record your thoughts, insights, and questions; your emotional outlook and physical state; and your successes and challenges.

_____

_____

_____

### Record everything you consume, including food, snacks, supplements, water, mints, and gum.

**Breakfast**

Water:

Supplements:

Morning snack:

**Lunch**

Water:

Supplements:

Midday snack:

**Dinner**

Water:

Supplements:

Evening snack:

**Exercise**

**HEALING CODES: Do the Healing Codes exercise on page 189 in *Perfect Weight America*. Record your stress level as you rated it while doing the exercise.**

| Healing Codes (AM) | Beginning: | End: | 10 min. later: |
|---|---|---|---|
| Healing Codes (PM) | Beginning: | End: | 10 min. later: |

Did you meet your Phase II goals today? _____

Record your thoughts, insights, and questions; your emotional outlook and physical state; and your successes and challenges.

_____

_____

_____

## Record everything you consume, including food, snacks, supplements, water, mints, and gum.

**Breakfast**

Water:

Supplements:

Morning snack:

**Lunch**

Water:

Supplements:

Midday snack:

**Dinner**

Water:

Supplements:

Evening snack:

**Exercise**

**HEALING CODES:** Do the Healing Codes exercise on page 189 in *Perfect Weight America*. Record your stress level as you rated it while doing the exercise.

| Healing Codes (AM) | Beginning: | End: | 10 min. later: |
| Healing Codes (PM) | Beginning: | End: | 10 min. later: |

Did you meet your Phase II goals today? _____

Record your thoughts, insights, and questions; your emotional outlook and physical state; and your successes and challenges.

_____

_____

_____

### Record everything you consume, including food, snacks, supplements, water, mints, and gum.

**Breakfast**

Water:

Supplements:

Morning snack:

**Lunch**

Water:

Supplements:

Midday snack:

**Dinner**

Water:

Supplements:

Evening snack:

**Exercise**

**HEALING CODES: Do the Healing Codes exercise on page 189 in *Perfect Weight America*. Record your stress level as you rated it while doing the exercise.**

| Healing Codes (AM) | Beginning: | End: | 10 min. later: |
|---|---|---|---|
| Healing Codes (PM) | Beginning: | End: | 10 min. later: |

Did you meet your Phase II goals today? _____

Record your thoughts, insights, and questions; your emotional outlook and physical state; and your successes and challenges.

_____

_____

_____

# Phase II, Week 7, Day 48          Date: _____

| Record everything you consume, including food, snacks, supplements, water, mints, and gum. |
|---|

**Breakfast**

Water:

Supplements:

Morning snack:

**Lunch**

Water:

Supplements:

Midday snack:

**Dinner**

Water:

Supplements:

Evening snack:

**Exercise**

| HEALING CODES: Do the Healing Codes exercise on page 189 in *Perfect Weight America*. Record your stress level as you rated it while doing the exercise. | | | |
|---|---|---|---|
| Healing Codes (AM) | Beginning: | End: | 10 min. later: |
| Healing Codes (PM) | Beginning: | End: | 10 min. later: |

Did you meet your Phase II goals today? _____

Record your thoughts, insights, and questions; your emotional outlook and physical state; and your successes and challenges.

_____

_____

_____

| Record everything you consume, including food, snacks, supplements, water, mints, and gum. |
| --- |

**Breakfast**


Water:
Supplements:
Morning snack:

**Lunch**


Water:
Supplements:
Midday snack:

**Dinner**


Water:
Supplements:
Evening snack:

**Exercise**


**HEALING CODES: Do the Healing Codes exercise on page 189 in *Perfect Weight America*. Record your stress level as you rated it while doing the exercise.**

| Healing Codes (AM) | Beginning: | End: | 10 min. later: |
| --- | --- | --- | --- |
| Healing Codes (PM) | Beginning: | End: | 10 min. later: |

Did you meet your Phase II goals today? _____

Record your thoughts, insights, and questions; your emotional outlook and physical state; and your successes and challenges.

_____

_____

_____

## Summary of Week 7

How many days did you follow the Perfect Weight Eating Plan? _____

How many days did you take the recommended supplements? _____

How many days did you drink at least half your body weight in ounces of water?

_____

How many days did you meet your goals for Phase II? _____

How many days did you exercise this week? _____

Write down any extra thoughts you want to capture about your week.

_____

_____

_____

_____

_____

_____

_____

_____

_____

_____

_____

_____

_____

_____

_____

_____

**Record everything you consume, including food, snacks, supplements, water, mints, and gum.**

**Breakfast**

Water:
Supplements:
Morning snack:

**Lunch**

Water:
Supplements:
Midday snack:

**Dinner**

Water:
Supplements:
Evening snack:

**Exercise**

**HEALING CODES: Do the Healing Codes exercise on page 189 in *Perfect Weight America*. Record your stress level as you rated it while doing the exercise.**

| Healing Codes (AM) | Beginning: | End: | 10 min. later: |
| Healing Codes (PM) | Beginning: | End: | 10 min. later: |

Did you meet your Phase II goals today? _____

Record your thoughts, insights, and questions; your emotional outlook and physical state; and your successes and challenges.

_____

_____

_____

| Record everything you consume, including food, snacks, supplements, water, mints, and gum. |
|---|

**Breakfast**




Water:
Supplements:
Morning snack:

**Lunch**




Water:
Supplements:
Midday snack:

**Dinner**




Water:
Supplements:
Evening snack:

**Exercise**


**HEALING CODES:** Do the Healing Codes exercise on page 189 in *Perfect Weight America*. Record your stress level as you rated it while doing the exercise.

| Healing Codes (AM) | Beginning: | End: | 10 min. later: |
|---|---|---|---|
| Healing Codes (PM) | Beginning: | End: | 10 min. later: |

Did you meet your Phase II goals today? _____

Record your thoughts, insights, and questions; your emotional outlook and physical state; and your successes and challenges.

_____

_____

_____

### Record everything you consume, including food, snacks, supplements, water, mints, and gum.

Breakfast

Water:
Supplements:
Morning snack:

Lunch

Water:
Supplements:
Midday snack:

Dinner

Water:
Supplements:
Evening snack:

Exercise

**HEALING CODES: Do the Healing Codes exercise on page 189 in *Perfect Weight America*. Record your stress level as you rated it while doing the exercise.**

| Healing Codes (AM) | Beginning: | End: | 10 min. later: |
| Healing Codes (PM) | Beginning: | End: | 10 min. later: |

Did you meet your Phase II goals today? _____

Record your thoughts, insights, and questions; your emotional outlook and physical state; and your successes and challenges.

_____

_____

_____

### Record everything you consume, including food, snacks, supplements, water, mints, and gum.

**Breakfast**

Water:

Supplements:

Morning snack:

**Lunch**

Water:

Supplements:

Midday snack:

**Dinner**

Water:

Supplements:

Evening snack:

**Exercise**

**HEALING CODES:** Do the Healing Codes exercise on page 189 in *Perfect Weight America*. Record your stress level as you rated it while doing the exercise.

| Healing Codes (AM) | Beginning: | End: | 10 min. later: |
| Healing Codes (PM) | Beginning: | End: | 10 min. later: |

Did you meet your Phase II goals today? _____

Record your thoughts, insights, and questions; your emotional outlook and physical state; and your successes and challenges.

**Record everything you consume, including food, snacks, supplements, water, mints, and gum.**

Breakfast

Water:
Supplements:
Morning snack:

Lunch

Water:
Supplements:
Midday snack:

Dinner

Water:
Supplements:
Evening snack:

Exercise

**HEALING CODES: Do the Healing Codes exercise on page 189 in *Perfect Weight America*. Record your stress level as you rated it while doing the exercise.**

| Healing Codes (AM) | Beginning: | End: | 10 min. later: |
| Healing Codes (PM) | Beginning: | End: | 10 min. later: |

Did you meet your Phase II goals today? _____

Record your thoughts, insights, and questions; your emotional outlook and physical state; and your successes and challenges.

_____

_____

_____

**Record everything you consume, including food, snacks, supplements, water, mints, and gum.**

### Breakfast

Water:
Supplements:
Morning snack:

### Lunch

Water:
Supplements:
Midday snack:

### Dinner

Water:
Supplements:
Evening snack:

### Exercise

**HEALING CODES:** Do the Healing Codes exercise on page 189 in *Perfect Weight America*. Record your stress level as you rated it while doing the exercise.

| Healing Codes (AM) | Beginning: | End: | 10 min. later: |
|---|---|---|---|
| Healing Codes (PM) | Beginning: | End: | 10 min. later: |

Did you meet your Phase II goals today? _____

Record your thoughts, insights, and questions; your emotional outlook and physical state; and your successes and challenges.

_____

_____

_____

| Record everything you consume, including food, snacks, supplements, water, mints, and gum. |
| --- |

**Breakfast**



Water:
Supplements:
Morning snack:

**Lunch**



Water:
Supplements:
Midday snack:

**Dinner**



Water:
Supplements:
Evening snack:

**Exercise**


| HEALING CODES: Do the Healing Codes exercise on page 189 in *Perfect Weight America*. Record your stress level as you rated it while doing the exercise. | | | |
| --- | --- | --- | --- |
| Healing Codes (AM) | Beginning: | End: | 10 min. later: |
| Healing Codes (PM) | Beginning: | End: | 10 min. later: |

Did you meet your Phase II goals today? _____

Record your thoughts, insights, and questions; your emotional outlook and physical state; and your successes and challenges.

_____

_____

_____

## Summary of Week 8

How many days did you follow the Perfect Weight Eating Plan? _____

How many days did you take the recommended supplements? _____

How many days did you drink at least half your body weight in ounces of water?

_____

How many days did you meet your goals for Phase II? _____

How many days did you exercise this week? _____

Write down any extra thoughts you want to capture about your week.

_____

_____

_____

_____

_____

_____

_____

_____

_____

_____

_____

_____

_____

_____

_____

_____

_____

## Phase III Goals

I will continue the progress I made in Phases I and II.

### Food and Beverage

I will add the following foods to my eating (see page 125 of *Perfect Weight America* for a complete list of allowed foods):

_____

_____

_____

I will avoid eating the following foods (see page 125 of *Perfect Weight America* for a complete list of foods to avoid):

_____

_____

_____

I will drink _____ ounces of water daily.

I will avoid drinking the following beverages:

_____

_____

_____

I will add the following healthy snacks to my daily snacking regimen:

_____

_____

_____

_____

## Phase III Goals

I will avoid the following snack foods:

_____

_____

### Supplements

I will take the following supplements daily:

_____

_____

### Exercise and Fitness Goals

I will do the following exercises at least four to five times a week:

_____

_____

_____

### Rest

I will go to bed by _____ each night.

### Other Goals for Phase III

_____

_____

_____

_____

_____

_____

**Record everything you consume, including food, snacks, supplements, water, mints, and gum.**

**Breakfast**

Water:
Supplements:
Morning snack:

**Lunch**

Water:
Supplements:
Midday snack:

**Dinner**

Water:
Supplements:
Evening snack:

**Exercise**

**HEALING CODES: Do the Healing Codes exercise on page 189 in *Perfect Weight America*. Record your stress level as you rated it while doing the exercise.**

| Healing Codes (AM) | Beginning: | End: | 10 min. later: |
| Healing Codes (PM) | Beginning: | End: | 10 min. later: |

Did you meet your Phase III goals today?_____

Record your thoughts, insights, and questions; your emotional outlook and physical state; and your successes and challenges.

_____

_____

_____

| Record everything you consume, including food, snacks, supplements, water, mints, and gum. |
|---|

**Breakfast**

Water:
Supplements:
Morning snack:

**Lunch**

Water:
Supplements:
Midday snack:

**Dinner**

Water:
Supplements:
Evening snack:

**Exercise**

**HEALING CODES: Do the Healing Codes exercise on page 189 in *Perfect Weight America*. Record your stress level as you rated it while doing the exercise.**

| Healing Codes (AM) | Beginning: | End: | 10 min. later: |
|---|---|---|---|
| Healing Codes (PM) | Beginning: | End: | 10 min. later: |

Did you meet your Phase III goals today? _____

Record your thoughts, insights, and questions; your emotional outlook and physical state; and your successes and challenges.

_____

_____

_____

**Record everything you consume, including food, snacks, supplements, water, mints, and gum.**

**Breakfast**

---

Water:
Supplements:
Morning snack:

**Lunch**

---

Water:
Supplements:
Midday snack:

**Dinner**

---

Water:
Supplements:
Evening snack:

**Exercise**

---

**HEALING CODES: Do the Healing Codes exercise on page 189 in *Perfect Weight America*. Record your stress level as you rated it while doing the exercise.**

| Healing Codes (AM) | Beginning: | End: | 10 min. later: |
| Healing Codes (PM) | Beginning: | End: | 10 min. later: |

Did you meet your Phase III goals today?_____

Record your thoughts, insights, and questions; your emotional outlook and physical state; and your successes and challenges.

---

---

---

## Record everything you consume, including food, snacks, supplements, water, mints, and gum.

**Breakfast**

Water:
Supplements:
Morning snack:

**Lunch**

Water:
Supplements:
Midday snack:

**Dinner**

Water:
Supplements:
Evening snack:

**Exercise**

**HEALING CODES: Do the Healing Codes exercise on page 189 in *Perfect Weight America*. Record your stress level as you rated it while doing the exercise.**

| Healing Codes (AM) | Beginning: | End: | 10 min. later: |
| Healing Codes (PM) | Beginning: | End: | 10 min. later: |

Did you meet your Phase III goals today? _____

Record your thoughts, insights, and questions; your emotional outlook and physical state; and your successes and challenges.

## Record everything you consume, including food, snacks, supplements, water, mints, and gum.

**Breakfast**

Water:

Supplements:

Morning snack:

**Lunch**

Water:

Supplements:

Midday snack:

**Dinner**

Water:

Supplements:

Evening snack:

**Exercise**

**HEALING CODES: Do the Healing Codes exercise on page 189 in *Perfect Weight America*. Record your stress level as you rated it while doing the exercise.**

| Healing Codes (AM) | Beginning: | End: | 10 min. later: |
| Healing Codes (PM) | Beginning: | End: | 10 min. later: |

Did you meet your Phase III goals today? _____

Record your thoughts, insights, and questions; your emotional outlook and physical state; and your successes and challenges.

_____

_____

_____

### Record everything you consume, including food, snacks, supplements, water, mints, and gum.

**Breakfast**

Water:
Supplements:
Morning snack:

**Lunch**

Water:
Supplements:
Midday snack:

**Dinner**

Water:
Supplements:
Evening snack:

**Exercise**

**HEALING CODES:** Do the Healing Codes exercise on page 189 in *Perfect Weight America*. Record your stress level as you rated it while doing the exercise.

| Healing Codes (AM) | Beginning: | End: | 10 min. later: |
| Healing Codes (PM) | Beginning: | End: | 10 min. later: |

Did you meet your Phase III goals today? _____

Record your thoughts, insights, and questions; your emotional outlook and physical state; and your successes and challenges.

_____

_____

_____

### Record everything you consume, including food, snacks, supplements, water, mints, and gum.

**Breakfast**

Water:
Supplements:
Morning snack:

**Lunch**

Water:
Supplements:
Midday snack:

**Dinner**

Water:
Supplements:
Evening snack:

**Exercise**

**HEALING CODES:** Do the Healing Codes exercise on page 189 in *Perfect Weight America*. Record your stress level as you rated it while doing the exercise.

| Healing Codes (AM) | Beginning: | End: | 10 min. later: |
| Healing Codes (PM) | Beginning: | End: | 10 min. later: |

Did you meet your Phase III goals today?_____

Record your thoughts, insights, and questions; your emotional outlook and physical state; and your successes and challenges.

_____

_____

_____

# Summary of Week 9

How many days did you follow the Perfect Weight Eating Plan? _____

How many days did you take the recommended supplements? _____

How many days did you drink at least half your body weight in ounces of water?

_____

How many days did you meet your goals for Phase III? _____

How many days did you exercise this week? _____

Write down any extra thoughts you want to capture about your week.

_____

_____

_____

_____

_____

_____

_____

_____

_____

_____

_____

_____

_____

_____

_____

_____

**Record everything you consume, including food, snacks, supplements, water, mints, and gum.**

**Breakfast**

Water:
Supplements:
Morning snack:

**Lunch**

Water:
Supplements:
Midday snack:

**Dinner**

Water:
Supplements:
Evening snack:

**Exercise**

**HEALING CODES: Do the Healing Codes exercise on page 189 in *Perfect Weight America*. Record your stress level as you rated it while doing the exercise.**

| Healing Codes (AM) | Beginning: | End: | 10 min. later: |
| Healing Codes (PM) | Beginning: | End: | 10 min. later: |

Did you meet your Phase III goals today? _____

Record your thoughts, insights, and questions; your emotional outlook and physical state; and your successes and challenges.

_____

_____

_____

| Record everything you consume, including food, snacks, supplements, water, mints, and gum. |
|---|

**Breakfast**




Water:
Supplements:
Morning snack:

**Lunch**




Water:
Supplements:
Midday snack:

**Dinner**




Water:
Supplements:
Evening snack:

**Exercise**


**HEALING CODES: Do the Healing Codes exercise on page 189 in _Perfect Weight America_. Record your stress level as you rated it while doing the exercise.**

| Healing Codes (AM) | Beginning: | End: | 10 min. later: |
|---|---|---|---|
| Healing Codes (PM) | Beginning: | End: | 10 min. later: |

Did you meet your Phase III goals today? _____

Record your thoughts, insights, and questions; your emotional outlook and physical state; and your successes and challenges.

_____

_____

_____

**Record everything you consume, including food, snacks, supplements, water, mints, and gum.**

### Breakfast

Water:
Supplements:
Morning snack:

### Lunch

Water:
Supplements:
Midday snack:

### Dinner

Water:
Supplements:
Evening snack:

### Exercise

**HEALING CODES: Do the Healing Codes exercise on page 189 in *Perfect Weight America*. Record your stress level as you rated it while doing the exercise.**

| Healing Codes (AM) | Beginning: | End: | 10 min. later: |
| Healing Codes (PM) | Beginning: | End: | 10 min. later: |

Did you meet your Phase III goals today? _____

Record your thoughts, insights, and questions; your emotional outlook and physical state; and your successes and challenges.

_____

_____

_____

| Record everything you consume, including food, snacks, supplements, water, mints, and gum. |
|---|

**Breakfast**

Water:
Supplements:
Morning snack:

**Lunch**

Water:
Supplements:
Midday snack:

**Dinner**

Water:
Supplements:
Evening snack:

**Exercise**

**HEALING CODES:** Do the Healing Codes exercise on page 189 in *Perfect Weight America*. Record your stress level as you rated it while doing the exercise.

| Healing Codes (AM) | Beginning: | End: | 10 min. later: |
|---|---|---|---|
| Healing Codes (PM) | Beginning: | End: | 10 min. later: |

Did you meet your Phase III goals today? _____

Record your thoughts, insights, and questions; your emotional outlook and physical state; and your successes and challenges.

_____

_____

_____

## Record everything you consume, including food, snacks, supplements, water, mints, and gum.

**Breakfast**

Water:
Supplements:
Morning snack:

**Lunch**

Water:
Supplements:
Midday snack:

**Dinner**

Water:
Supplements:
Evening snack:

**Exercise**

**HEALING CODES: Do the Healing Codes exercise on page 189 in *Perfect Weight America*. Record your stress level as you rated it while doing the exercise.**

| Healing Codes (AM) | Beginning: | End: | 10 min. later: |
| Healing Codes (PM) | Beginning: | End: | 10 min. later: |

Did you meet your Phase III goals today? _____

Record your thoughts, insights, and questions; your emotional outlook and physical state; and your successes and challenges.

_____

_____

_____

**Record everything you consume, including food, snacks, supplements, water, mints, and gum.**

Breakfast

Water:
Supplements:
Morning snack:

Lunch

Water:
Supplements:
Midday snack:

Dinner

Water:
Supplements:
Evening snack:

Exercise

**HEALING CODES: Do the Healing Codes exercise on page 189 in *Perfect Weight America*. Record your stress level as you rated it while doing the exercise.**

| Healing Codes (AM) | Beginning: | End: | 10 min. later: |
| Healing Codes (PM) | Beginning: | End: | 10 min. later: |

Did you meet your Phase III goals today? _____

Record your thoughts, insights, and questions; your emotional outlook and physical state; and your successes and challenges.

_____

_____

_____

**Record everything you consume, including food, snacks, supplements, water, mints, and gum.**

### Breakfast

Water:

Supplements:

Morning snack:

### Lunch

Water:

Supplements:

Midday snack:

### Dinner

Water:

Supplements:

Evening snack:

### Exercise

**HEALING CODES: Do the Healing Codes exercise on page 189 in *Perfect Weight America*. Record your stress level as you rated it while doing the exercise.**

| Healing Codes (AM) | Beginning: | End: | 10 min. later: |
| Healing Codes (PM) | Beginning: | End: | 10 min. later: |

Did you meet your Phase III goals today? _____

Record your thoughts, insights, and questions; your emotional outlook and physical state; and your successes and challenges.

_____

_____

_____

## Summary of Week 10

How many days did you follow the Perfect Weight Eating Plan? _____

How many days did you take the recommended supplements? _____

How many days did you drink at least half your body weight in ounces of water?

_____

How many days did you meet your goals for Phase III? _____

How many days did you exercise this week? _____

Write down any extra thoughts you want to capture about your week.

_____

_____

_____

_____

_____

_____

_____

_____

_____

_____

_____

_____

_____

_____

**Record everything you consume, including food, snacks, supplements, water, mints, and gum.**

Breakfast

Water:
Supplements:
Morning snack:

Lunch

Water:
Supplements:
Midday snack:

Dinner

Water:
Supplements:
Evening snack:

Exercise

**HEALING CODES: Do the Healing Codes exercise on page 189 in *Perfect Weight America*. Record your stress level as you rated it while doing the exercise.**

| Healing Codes (AM) | Beginning: | End: | 10 min. later: |
| Healing Codes (PM) | Beginning: | End: | 10 min. later: |

Did you meet your Phase III goals today? _____

Record your thoughts, insights, and questions; your emotional outlook and physical state; and your successes and challenges.

_____

_____

_____

**Record everything you consume, including food, snacks, supplements, water, mints, and gum.**

**Breakfast**

Water:
Supplements:
Morning snack:

**Lunch**

Water:
Supplements:
Midday snack:

**Dinner**

Water:
Supplements:
Evening snack:

**Exercise**

**HEALING CODES:** Do the Healing Codes exercise on page 189 in *Perfect Weight America*. Record your stress level as you rated it while doing the exercise.

| Healing Codes (AM) | Beginning: | End: | 10 min. later: |
| Healing Codes (PM) | Beginning: | End: | 10 min. later: |

Did you meet your Phase III goals today?_____

Record your thoughts, insights, and questions; your emotional outlook and physical state; and your successes and challenges.

_____

_____

_____

**Record everything you consume, including food, snacks, supplements, water, mints, and gum.**

**Breakfast**

Water:
Supplements:
Morning snack:

**Lunch**

Water:
Supplements:
Midday snack:

**Dinner**

Water:
Supplements:
Evening snack:

**Exercise**

**HEALING CODES: Do the Healing Codes exercise on page 189 in *Perfect Weight America*. Record your stress level as you rated it while doing the exercise.**

| Healing Codes (AM) | Beginning: | End: | 10 min. later: |
| Healing Codes (PM) | Beginning: | End: | 10 min. later: |

Did you meet your Phase III goals today? _____

Record your thoughts, insights, and questions; your emotional outlook and physical state; and your successes and challenges.

_____

_____

_____

## Record everything you consume, including food, snacks, supplements, water, mints, and gum.

**Breakfast**

Water:
Supplements:
Morning snack:

**Lunch**

Water:
Supplements:
Midday snack:

**Dinner**

Water:
Supplements:
Evening snack:

**Exercise**

**HEALING CODES:** Do the Healing Codes exercise on page 189 in *Perfect Weight America*. Record your stress level as you rated it while doing the exercise.

| Healing Codes (AM) | Beginning: | End: | 10 min. later: |
|---|---|---|---|
| Healing Codes (PM) | Beginning: | End: | 10 min. later: |

Did you meet your Phase III goals today? _____

Record your thoughts, insights, and questions; your emotional outlook and physical state; and your successes and challenges.

_____

_____

_____

| Record everything you consume, including food, snacks, supplements, water, mints, and gum. |
|---|

**Breakfast**



Water:
Supplements:
Morning snack:

**Lunch**



Water:
Supplements:
Midday snack:

**Dinner**



Water:
Supplements:
Evening snack:

**Exercise**


**HEALING CODES:** Do the Healing Codes exercise on page 189 in *Perfect Weight America*. Record your stress level as you rated it while doing the exercise.

| Healing Codes (AM) | Beginning: | End: | 10 min. later: |
|---|---|---|---|
| Healing Codes (PM) | Beginning: | End: | 10 min. later: |

Did you meet your Phase III goals today? _____

Record your thoughts, insights, and questions; your emotional outlook and physical state; and your successes and challenges.

_____

_____

_____

| Record everything you consume, including food, snacks, supplements, water, mints, and gum. |
|---|

**Breakfast**

Water:

Supplements:

Morning snack:

**Lunch**

Water:

Supplements:

Midday snack:

**Dinner**

Water:

Supplements:

Evening snack:

**Exercise**

**HEALING CODES:** Do the Healing Codes exercise on page 189 in *Perfect Weight America*. Record your stress level as you rated it while doing the exercise.

| Healing Codes (AM) | Beginning: | End: | 10 min. later: |
|---|---|---|---|
| Healing Codes (PM) | Beginning: | End: | 10 min. later: |

Did you meet your Phase III goals today? _____

Record your thoughts, insights, and questions; your emotional outlook and physical state; and your successes and challenges.

_____

_____

_____

### Record everything you consume, including food, snacks, supplements, water, mints, and gum.

**Breakfast**

Water:

Supplements:

Morning snack:

**Lunch**

Water:

Supplements:

Midday snack:

**Dinner**

Water:

Supplements:

Evening snack:

**Exercise**

**HEALING CODES: Do the Healing Codes exercise on page 189 in *Perfect Weight America*. Record your stress level as you rated it while doing the exercise.**

| Healing Codes (AM) | Beginning: | End: | 10 min. later: |
|---|---|---|---|
| Healing Codes (PM) | Beginning: | End: | 10 min. later: |

Did you meet your Phase III goals today? _____

Record your thoughts, insights, and questions; your emotional outlook and physical state; and your successes and challenges.

_____

_____

_____

# Summary of Week 11

How many days did you follow the Perfect Weight Eating Plan? _____

How many days did you take the recommended supplements? _____

How many days did you drink at least half your body weight in ounces of water?

_____

How many days did you meet your goals for Phase III? _____

How many days did you exercise this week? _____

Write down any extra thoughts you want to capture about your week.

_____

_____

_____

_____

_____

_____

_____

_____

_____

_____

_____

_____

_____

_____

**Record everything you consume, including food, snacks, supplements, water, mints, and gum.**

**Breakfast**

Water:

Supplements:

Morning snack:

**Lunch**

Water:

Supplements:

Midday snack:

**Dinner**

Water:

Supplements:

Evening snack:

**Exercise**

**HEALING CODES: Do the Healing Codes exercise on page 189 in *Perfect Weight America*. Record your stress level as you rated it while doing the exercise.**

| Healing Codes (AM) | Beginning: | End: | 10 min. later: |
|---|---|---|---|
| Healing Codes (PM) | Beginning: | End: | 10 min. later: |

Did you meet your Phase III goals today? _____

Record your thoughts, insights, and questions; your emotional outlook and physical state; and your successes and challenges.

_____

_____

_____

| Record everything you consume, including food, snacks, supplements, water, mints, and gum. |
|---|

**Breakfast**

Water:
Supplements:
Morning snack:

**Lunch**

Water:
Supplements:
Midday snack:

**Dinner**

Water:
Supplements:
Evening snack:

**Exercise**

**HEALING CODES: Do the Healing Codes exercise on page 189 in _Perfect Weight America_. Record your stress level as you rated it while doing the exercise.**

| Healing Codes (AM) | Beginning: | End: | 10 min. later: |
|---|---|---|---|
| Healing Codes (PM) | Beginning: | End: | 10 min. later: |

Did you meet your Phase III goals today? _____

Record your thoughts, insights, and questions; your emotional outlook and physical state; and your successes and challenges.

_____

_____

_____

**Record everything you consume, including food, snacks, supplements, water, mints, and gum.**

Breakfast

Water:
Supplements:
Morning snack:

Lunch

Water:
Supplements:
Midday snack:

Dinner

Water:
Supplements:
Evening snack:

Exercise

**HEALING CODES: Do the Healing Codes exercise on page 189 in *Perfect Weight America*. Record your stress level as you rated it while doing the exercise.**

| Healing Codes (AM) | Beginning: | End: | 10 min. later: |
|---|---|---|---|
| Healing Codes (PM) | Beginning: | End: | 10 min. later: |

Did you meet your Phase III goals today? _____

Record your thoughts, insights, and questions; your emotional outlook and physical state; and your successes and challenges.

_____

_____

_____

| Record everything you consume, including food, snacks, supplements, water, mints, and gum. |
|---|

**Breakfast**

Water:
Supplements:
Morning snack:

**Lunch**

Water:
Supplements:
Midday snack:

**Dinner**

Water:
Supplements:
Evening snack:

**Exercise**

**HEALING CODES:** Do the Healing Codes exercise on page 189 in *Perfect Weight America*. Record your stress level as you rated it while doing the exercise.

| Healing Codes (AM) | Beginning: | End: | 10 min. later: |
|---|---|---|---|
| Healing Codes (PM) | Beginning: | End: | 10 min. later: |

Did you meet your Phase III goals today? _____

Record your thoughts, insights, and questions; your emotional outlook and physical state; and your successes and challenges.

**Record everything you consume, including food, snacks, supplements, water, mints, and gum.**

**Breakfast**

Water:
Supplements:
Morning snack:

**Lunch**

Water:
Supplements:
Midday snack:

**Dinner**

Water:
Supplements:
Evening snack:

**Exercise**

**HEALING CODES: Do the Healing Codes exercise on page 189 in *Perfect Weight America*. Record your stress level as you rated it while doing the exercise.**

| Healing Codes (AM) | Beginning: | End: | 10 min. later: |
| Healing Codes (PM) | Beginning: | End: | 10 min. later: |

Did you meet your Phase III goals today? _____

Record your thoughts, insights, and questions; your emotional outlook and physical state; and your successes and challenges.

_____

_____

_____

| Record everything you consume, including food, snacks, supplements, water, mints, and gum. |
|---|

**Breakfast**



Water:
Supplements:
Morning snack:

**Lunch**



Water:
Supplements:
Midday snack:

**Dinner**



Water:
Supplements:
Evening snack:

**Exercise**


**HEALING CODES: Do the Healing Codes exercise on page 189 in *Perfect Weight America*. Record your stress level as you rated it while doing the exercise.**

| Healing Codes (AM) | Beginning: | End: | 10 min. later: |
|---|---|---|---|
| Healing Codes (PM) | Beginning: | End: | 10 min. later: |

Did you meet your Phase III goals today? _____

Record your thoughts, insights, and questions; your emotional outlook and physical state; and your successes and challenges.

_____

_____

_____

| Record everything you consume, including food, snacks, supplements, water, mints, and gum. |
| --- |

**Breakfast**

Water:
Supplements:
Morning snack:

**Lunch**

Water:
Supplements:
Midday snack:

**Dinner**

Water:
Supplements:
Evening snack:

**Exercise**

**HEALING CODES:** Do the Healing Codes exercise on page 189 in *Perfect Weight America*. Record your stress level as you rated it while doing the exercise.

| Healing Codes (AM) | Beginning: | End: | 10 min. later: |
| --- | --- | --- | --- |
| Healing Codes (PM) | Beginning: | End: | 10 min. later: |

Did you meet your Phase III goals today? _____

Record your thoughts, insights, and questions; your emotional outlook and physical state; and your successes and challenges.

_____

_____

_____

# Summary of Week 12

How many days did you follow the Perfect Weight Eating Plan? _____

How many days did you take the recommended supplements? _____

How many days did you drink at least half your body weight in ounces of water?

_____

How many days did you meet your goals for Phase III? _____

How many days did you exercise this week? _____

Write down any extra thoughts you want to capture about your week.

_____

_____

_____

_____

_____

_____

_____

_____

_____

_____

_____

_____

_____

_____

_____

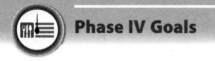

# Phase IV Goals

I will continue the progress I made in Phases I, II, and III.

## Food and Beverage

I will add the following foods to my eating (see page 126 of *Perfect Weight America* for a complete list of allowed foods):

_____

_____

_____

I will avoid eating the following foods (see page 126 of *Perfect Weight America* for a complete list of foods to avoid):

_____

_____

_____

I will drink _____ ounces of water daily.

I will avoid drinking the following beverages:

_____

_____

_____

I will add the following healthy snacks to my daily snacking regimen:

_____

_____

_____

_____

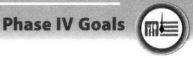

I will avoid the following snack foods:

_____

_____

## Supplements

I will take the following supplements daily:

_____

_____

## Exercise and Fitness Goals

I will do the following exercises at least four to five times a week:

_____

_____

_____

## Rest

I will go to bed by _____ each night.

## Other Goals for Phase IV

_____

_____

_____

_____

_____

_____

**Record everything you consume, including food, snacks, supplements, water, mints, and gum.**

**Breakfast**

Water:

Supplements:

Morning snack:

**Lunch**

Water:

Supplements:

Midday snack:

**Dinner**

Water:

Supplements:

Evening snack:

**Exercise**

**HEALING CODES: Do the Healing Codes exercise on page 189 in *Perfect Weight America*. Record your stress level as you rated it while doing the exercise.**

| Healing Codes (AM) | Beginning: | End: | 10 min. later: |
| Healing Codes (PM) | Beginning: | End: | 10 min. later: |

Did you meet your Phase IV goals today? _____

Record your thoughts, insights, and questions; your emotional outlook and physical state; and your successes and challenges.

_____

_____

_____

## Record everything you consume, including food, snacks, supplements, water, mints, and gum.

**Breakfast**

Water:
Supplements:
Morning snack:

**Lunch**

Water:
Supplements:
Midday snack:

**Dinner**

Water:
Supplements:
Evening snack:

**Exercise**

**HEALING CODES:** Do the Healing Codes exercise on page 189 in *Perfect Weight America*. Record your stress level as you rated it while doing the exercise.

| Healing Codes (AM) | Beginning: | End: | 10 min. later: |
| Healing Codes (PM) | Beginning: | End: | 10 min. later: |

Did you meet your Phase IV goals today? _____

Record your thoughts, insights, and questions; your emotional outlook and physical state; and your successes and challenges.

_____

_____

_____

**Record everything you consume, including food, snacks, supplements, water, mints, and gum.**

**Breakfast**



Water:
Supplements:
Morning snack:

**Lunch**



Water:
Supplements:
Midday snack:

**Dinner**



Water:
Supplements:
Evening snack:

**Exercise**


**HEALING CODES: Do the Healing Codes exercise on page 189 in *Perfect Weight America*. Record your stress level as you rated it while doing the exercise.**

| Healing Codes (AM) | Beginning: | End: | 10 min. later: |
| Healing Codes (PM) | Beginning: | End: | 10 min. later: |

Did you meet your Phase IV goals today? _____

Record your thoughts, insights, and questions; your emotional outlook and physical state; and your successes and challenges.

_____

_____

_____

**Record everything you consume, including food, snacks, supplements, water, mints, and gum.**

Breakfast

Water:
Supplements:
Morning snack:

Lunch

Water:
Supplements:
Midday snack:

Dinner

Water:
Supplements:
Evening snack:

Exercise

**HEALING CODES: Do the Healing Codes exercise on page 189 in *Perfect Weight America*. Record your stress level as you rated it while doing the exercise.**

| Healing Codes (AM) | Beginning: | End: | 10 min. later: |
| Healing Codes (PM) | Beginning: | End: | 10 min. later: |

Did you meet your Phase IV goals today? _____

Record your thoughts, insights, and questions; your emotional outlook and physical state; and your successes and challenges.

_____

_____

_____

**Record everything you consume, including food, snacks, supplements, water, mints, and gum.**

Breakfast

Water:
Supplements:
Morning snack:

Lunch

Water:
Supplements:
Midday snack:

Dinner

Water:
Supplements:
Evening snack:

Exercise

**HEALING CODES: Do the Healing Codes exercise on page 189 in *Perfect Weight America*. Record your stress level as you rated it while doing the exercise.**

| Healing Codes (AM) | Beginning: | End: | 10 min. later: |
| Healing Codes (PM) | Beginning: | End: | 10 min. later: |

Did you meet your Phase IV goals today? _____

Record your thoughts, insights, and questions; your emotional outlook and physical state; and your successes and challenges.

_____

_____

_____

**Record everything you consume, including food, snacks, supplements, water, mints, and gum.**

**Breakfast**



Water:
Supplements:
Morning snack:

**Lunch**



Water:
Supplements:
Midday snack:

**Dinner**



Water:
Supplements:
Evening snack:

**Exercise**


**HEALING CODES: Do the Healing Codes exercise on page 189 in *Perfect Weight America*. Record your stress level as you rated it while doing the exercise.**

| Healing Codes (AM) | Beginning: | End: | 10 min. later: |
| Healing Codes (PM) | Beginning: | End: | 10 min. later: |

Did you meet your Phase IV goals today? _____

Record your thoughts, insights, and questions; your emotional outlook and physical state; and your successes and challenges.

_____

_____

_____

**Record everything you consume, including food, snacks, supplements, water, mints, and gum.**

**Breakfast**

Water:

Supplements:

Morning snack:

**Lunch**

Water:

Supplements:

Midday snack:

**Dinner**

Water:

Supplements:

Evening snack:

**Exercise**

**HEALING CODES: Do the Healing Codes exercise on page 189 in *Perfect Weight America*. Record your stress level as you rated it while doing the exercise.**

| Healing Codes (AM) | Beginning: | End: | 10 min. later: |
| --- | --- | --- | --- |
| Healing Codes (PM) | Beginning: | End: | 10 min. later: |

Did you meet your Phase IV goals today? _____

Record your thoughts, insights, and questions; your emotional outlook and physical state; and your successes and challenges.

_____

_____

_____

# Summary of Week 13

How many days did you follow the Perfect Weight Eating Plan? _____

How many days did you take the recommended supplements? _____

How many days did you drink at least half your body weight in ounces of water?

_____

How many days did you meet your goals for Phase IV? _____

How many days did you exercise this week? _____

Write down any extra thoughts you want to capture about your week.

_____

_____

_____

_____

_____

_____

_____

_____

_____

_____

_____

_____

_____

_____

**Record everything you consume, including food, snacks, supplements, water, mints, and gum.**

Breakfast

Water:
Supplements:
Morning snack:

Lunch

Water:
Supplements:
Midday snack:

Dinner

Water:
Supplements:
Evening snack:

Exercise

**HEALING CODES: Do the Healing Codes exercise on page 189 in *Perfect Weight America*. Record your stress level as you rated it while doing the exercise.**

| Healing Codes (AM) | Beginning: | End: | 10 min. later: |
| Healing Codes (PM) | Beginning: | End: | 10 min. later: |

Did you meet your Phase IV goals today? _____

Record your thoughts, insights, and questions; your emotional outlook and physical state; and your successes and challenges.

_____

_____

_____

## Record everything you consume, including food, snacks, supplements, water, mints, and gum.

**Breakfast**

Water:
Supplements:
Morning snack:

**Lunch**

Water:
Supplements:
Midday snack:

**Dinner**

Water:
Supplements:
Evening snack:

**Exercise**

**HEALING CODES:** Do the Healing Codes exercise on page 189 in *Perfect Weight America*. Record your stress level as you rated it while doing the exercise.

| Healing Codes (AM) | Beginning: | End: | 10 min. later: |
| Healing Codes (PM) | Beginning: | End: | 10 min. later: |

Did you meet your Phase IV goals today? _____

Record your thoughts, insights, and questions; your emotional outlook and physical state; and your successes and challenges.

_____

_____

_____

**Record everything you consume, including food, snacks, supplements, water, mints, and gum.**

**Breakfast**

Water:

Supplements:

Morning snack:

**Lunch**

Water:

Supplements:

Midday snack:

**Dinner**

Water:

Supplements:

Evening snack:

**Exercise**

**HEALING CODES: Do the Healing Codes exercise on page 189 in *Perfect Weight America*. Record your stress level as you rated it while doing the exercise.**

| Healing Codes (AM) | Beginning: | End: | 10 min. later: |
| Healing Codes (PM) | Beginning: | End: | 10 min. later: |

Did you meet your Phase IV goals today? _____

Record your thoughts, insights, and questions; your emotional outlook and physical state; and your successes and challenges.

_____

_____

_____

| Record everything you consume, including food, snacks, supplements, water, mints, and gum. |
|---|

**Breakfast**

---
---
---

Water:
Supplements:
Morning snack:

**Lunch**

---
---
---

Water:
Supplements:
Midday snack:

**Dinner**

---
---
---

Water:
Supplements:
Evening snack:

**Exercise**

---

| HEALING CODES: Do the Healing Codes exercise on page 189 in *Perfect Weight America*. Record your stress level as you rated it while doing the exercise. | | | |
|---|---|---|---|
| Healing Codes (AM) | Beginning: | End: | 10 min. later: |
| Healing Codes (PM) | Beginning: | End: | 10 min. later: |

Did you meet your Phase IV goals today? _____

Record your thoughts, insights, and questions; your emotional outlook and physical state; and your successes and challenges.

---
---
---

| Record everything you consume, including food, snacks, supplements, water, mints, and gum. |
| --- |

**Breakfast**



Water:
Supplements:
Morning snack:

**Lunch**



Water:
Supplements:
Midday snack:

**Dinner**



Water:
Supplements:
Evening snack:

**Exercise**


| HEALING CODES: Do the Healing Codes exercise on page 189 in *Perfect Weight America*. Record your stress level as you rated it while doing the exercise. | | | |
| --- | --- | --- | --- |
| Healing Codes (AM) | Beginning: | End: | 10 min. later: |
| Healing Codes (PM) | Beginning: | End: | 10 min. later: |

Did you meet your Phase IV goals today? _____

Record your thoughts, insights, and questions; your emotional outlook and physical state; and your successes and challenges.

_____

_____

_____

| Record everything you consume, including food, snacks, supplements, water, mints, and gum. |
|---|

**Breakfast**

Water:
Supplements:
Morning snack:

**Lunch**

Water:
Supplements:
Midday snack:

**Dinner**

Water:
Supplements:
Evening snack:

**Exercise**

| HEALING CODES: Do the Healing Codes exercise on page 189 in *Perfect Weight America*. Record your stress level as you rated it while doing the exercise. | | | |
|---|---|---|---|
| Healing Codes (AM) | Beginning: | End: | 10 min. later: |
| Healing Codes (PM) | Beginning: | End: | 10 min. later: |

Did you meet your Phase IV goals today? _____

Record your thoughts, insights, and questions; your emotional outlook and physical state; and your successes and challenges.

_____

_____

_____

**Record everything you consume, including food, snacks, supplements, water, mints, and gum.**

Breakfast

Water:
Supplements:
Morning snack:

Lunch

Water:
Supplements:
Midday snack:

Dinner

Water:
Supplements:
Evening snack:

Exercise

**HEALING CODES: Do the Healing Codes exercise on page 189 in *Perfect Weight America*. Record your stress level as you rated it while doing the exercise.**

| Healing Codes (AM) | Beginning: | End: | 10 min. later: |
|---|---|---|---|
| Healing Codes (PM) | Beginning: | End: | 10 min. later: |

Did you meet your Phase IV goals today? _____

Record your thoughts, insights, and questions; your emotional outlook and physical state; and your successes and challenges.

_____

_____

_____

# Summary of Week 14

How many days did you follow the Perfect Weight Eating Plan? _____

How many days did you take the recommended supplements? _____

How many days did you drink at least half your body weight in ounces of water?

_____

How many days did you meet your goals for Phase IV? _____

How many days did you exercise this week? _____

Write down any extra thoughts you want to capture about your week.

_____

_____

_____

_____

_____

_____

_____

_____

_____

_____

_____

_____

_____

_____

_____

_____

## Record everything you consume, including food, snacks, supplements, water, mints, and gum.

**Breakfast**

Water:
Supplements:
Morning snack:

**Lunch**

Water:
Supplements:
Midday snack:

**Dinner**

Water:
Supplements:
Evening snack:

**Exercise**

**HEALING CODES:** Do the Healing Codes exercise on page 189 in *Perfect Weight America*. Record your stress level as you rated it while doing the exercise.

| Healing Codes (AM) | Beginning: | End: | 10 min. later: |
| Healing Codes (PM) | Beginning: | End: | 10 min. later: |

Did you meet your Phase IV goals today? _____

Record your thoughts, insights, and questions; your emotional outlook and physical state; and your successes and challenges.

| Record everything you consume, including food, snacks, supplements, water, mints, and gum. |
|---|

**Breakfast**
_____
_____
_____

Water:
Supplements:
Morning snack:

**Lunch**
_____
_____
_____

Water:
Supplements:
Midday snack:

**Dinner**
_____
_____
_____

Water:
Supplements:
Evening snack:

**Exercise**
_____

**HEALING CODES:** Do the Healing Codes exercise on page 189 in *Perfect Weight America*. Record your stress level as you rated it while doing the exercise.

| Healing Codes (AM) | Beginning: | End: | 10 min. later: |
|---|---|---|---|
| Healing Codes (PM) | Beginning: | End: | 10 min. later: |

Did you meet your Phase IV goals today? _____

Record your thoughts, insights, and questions; your emotional outlook and physical state; and your successes and challenges.

_____

_____

_____

**Record everything you consume, including food, snacks, supplements, water, mints, and gum.**

**Breakfast**

Water:
Supplements:
Morning snack:

**Lunch**

Water:
Supplements:
Midday snack:

**Dinner**

Water:
Supplements:
Evening snack:

**Exercise**

**HEALING CODES:** Do the Healing Codes exercise on page 189 in *Perfect Weight America*. Record your stress level as you rated it while doing the exercise.

| Healing Codes (AM) | Beginning: | End: | 10 min. later: |
| Healing Codes (PM) | Beginning: | End: | 10 min. later: |

Did you meet your Phase IV goals today? _____

Record your thoughts, insights, and questions; your emotional outlook and physical state; and your successes and challenges.

_____

_____

_____

## Record everything you consume, including food, snacks, supplements, water, mints, and gum.

**Breakfast**

Water:
Supplements:
Morning snack:

**Lunch**

Water:
Supplements:
Midday snack:

**Dinner**

Water:
Supplements:
Evening snack:

**Exercise**

**HEALING CODES:** Do the Healing Codes exercise on page 189 in *Perfect Weight America*. Record your stress level as you rated it while doing the exercise.

| Healing Codes (AM) | Beginning: | End: | 10 min. later: |
| Healing Codes (PM) | Beginning: | End: | 10 min. later: |

Did you meet your Phase IV goals today? _____

Record your thoughts, insights, and questions; your emotional outlook and physical state; and your successes and challenges.

_____

_____

_____

| Record everything you consume, including food, snacks, supplements, water, mints, and gum. |
| --- |

**Breakfast**




Water:
Supplements:
Morning snack:

**Lunch**




Water:
Supplements:
Midday snack:

**Dinner**




Water:
Supplements:
Evening snack:

**Exercise**


| HEALING CODES: Do the Healing Codes exercise on page 189 in *Perfect Weight America*. Record your stress level as you rated it while doing the exercise. | | | |
| --- | --- | --- | --- |
| Healing Codes (AM) | Beginning: | End: | 10 min. later: |
| Healing Codes (PM) | Beginning: | End: | 10 min. later: |

Did you meet your Phase IV goals today? _____

Record your thoughts, insights, and questions; your emotional outlook and physical state; and your successes and challenges.

_____

_____

_____

## Phase IV, Week 15, Day 104       Date: _____

**Record everything you consume, including food, snacks, supplements, water, mints, and gum.**

Breakfast
_____
_____
_____

Water:
Supplements:
Morning snack:

Lunch
_____
_____
_____

Water:
Supplements:
Midday snack:

Dinner
_____
_____
_____

Water:
Supplements:
Evening snack:

Exercise
_____

**HEALING CODES: Do the Healing Codes exercise on page 189 in *Perfect Weight America*. Record your stress level as you rated it while doing the exercise.**

| Healing Codes (AM) | Beginning: | End: | 10 min. later: |
| Healing Codes (PM) | Beginning: | End: | 10 min. later: |

Did you meet your Phase IV goals today? _____

Record your thoughts, insights, and questions; your emotional outlook and physical state; and your successes and challenges.

_____
_____
_____

**Record everything you consume, including food, snacks, supplements, water, mints, and gum.**

**Breakfast**

Water:
Supplements:
Morning snack:

**Lunch**

Water:
Supplements:
Midday snack:

**Dinner**

Water:
Supplements:
Evening snack:

**Exercise**

**HEALING CODES: Do the Healing Codes exercise on page 189 in *Perfect Weight America*. Record your stress level as you rated it while doing the exercise.**

| Healing Codes (AM) | Beginning: | End: | 10 min. later: |
|---|---|---|---|
| Healing Codes (PM) | Beginning: | End: | 10 min. later: |

Did you meet your Phase IV goals today? _____

Record your thoughts, insights, and questions; your emotional outlook and physical state; and your successes and challenges.

_____

_____

_____

## Summary of Week 15

How many days did you follow the Perfect Weight Eating Plan? _____

How many days did you take the recommended supplements? _____

How many days did you drink at least half your body weight in ounces of water?

_____

How many days did you meet your goals for Phase IV?_____

How many days did you exercise this week? _____

Write down any extra thoughts you want to capture about your week.

_____

_____

_____

_____

_____

_____

_____

_____

_____

_____

_____

_____

_____

_____

_____

### Record everything you consume, including food, snacks, supplements, water, mints, and gum.

**Breakfast**

Water:

Supplements:

Morning snack:

**Lunch**

Water:

Supplements:

Midday snack:

**Dinner**

Water:

Supplements:

Evening snack:

**Exercise**

**HEALING CODES:** Do the Healing Codes exercise on page 189 in *Perfect Weight America*. Record your stress level as you rated it while doing the exercise.

| Healing Codes (AM) | Beginning: | End: | 10 min. later: |
| Healing Codes (PM) | Beginning: | End: | 10 min. later: |

Did you meet your Phase IV goals today? _____

Record your thoughts, insights, and questions; your emotional outlook and physical state; and your successes and challenges.

| Record everything you consume, including food, snacks, supplements, water, mints, and gum. |
| --- |

**Breakfast**

Water:
Supplements:
Morning snack:

**Lunch**

Water:
Supplements:
Midday snack:

**Dinner**

Water:
Supplements:
Evening snack:

**Exercise**

| HEALING CODES: Do the Healing Codes exercise on page 189 in *Perfect Weight America*. Record your stress level as you rated it while doing the exercise. | | | |
| --- | --- | --- | --- |
| Healing Codes (AM) | Beginning: | End: | 10 min. later: |
| Healing Codes (PM) | Beginning: | End: | 10 min. later: |

Did you meet your Phase IV goals today? _____

Record your thoughts, insights, and questions; your emotional outlook and physical state; and your successes and challenges.

_____

_____

_____

### Record everything you consume, including food, snacks, supplements, water, mints, and gum.

**Breakfast**

Water:

Supplements:

Morning snack:

**Lunch**

Water:

Supplements:

Midday snack:

**Dinner**

Water:

Supplements:

Evening snack:

**Exercise**

**HEALING CODES: Do the Healing Codes exercise on page 189 in *Perfect Weight America*. Record your stress level as you rated it while doing the exercise.**

| Healing Codes (AM) | Beginning: | End: | 10 min. later: |
|---|---|---|---|
| Healing Codes (PM) | Beginning: | End: | 10 min. later: |

Did you meet your Phase IV goals today? _____

Record your thoughts, insights, and questions; your emotional outlook and physical state; and your successes and challenges.

_____

_____

_____

| Record everything you consume, including food, snacks, supplements, water, mints, and gum. |
|---|
| **Breakfast** |
| |
| |
| |
| Water: |
| Supplements: |
| Morning snack: |
| **Lunch** |
| |
| |
| |
| Water: |
| Supplements: |
| Midday snack: |
| **Dinner** |
| |
| |
| |
| Water: |
| Supplements: |
| Evening snack: |
| **Exercise** |
| |

| HEALING CODES: Do the Healing Codes exercise on page 189 in *Perfect Weight America*. Record your stress level as you rated it while doing the exercise. | | | |
|---|---|---|---|
| Healing Codes (AM) | Beginning: | End: | 10 min. later: |
| Healing Codes (PM) | Beginning: | End: | 10 min. later: |

Did you meet your Phase IV goals today? _____

Record your thoughts, insights, and questions; your emotional outlook and physical state; and your successes and challenges.

_____

_____

_____

## Record everything you consume, including food, snacks, supplements, water, mints, and gum.

**Breakfast**

Water:
Supplements:
Morning snack:

**Lunch**

Water:
Supplements:
Midday snack:

**Dinner**

Water:
Supplements:
Evening snack:

**Exercise**

## HEALING CODES: Do the Healing Codes exercise on page 189 in *Perfect Weight America*. Record your stress level as you rated it while doing the exercise.

| Healing Codes (AM) | Beginning: | End: | 10 min. later: |
| Healing Codes (PM) | Beginning: | End: | 10 min. later: |

Did you meet your Phase IV goals today? _____

Record your thoughts, insights, and questions; your emotional outlook and physical state; and your successes and challenges.

_____

_____

_____

| Record everything you consume, including food, snacks, supplements, water, mints, and gum. |
|---|

**Breakfast**

Water:
Supplements:
Morning snack:

**Lunch**

Water:
Supplements:
Midday snack:

**Dinner**

Water:
Supplements:
Evening snack:

**Exercise**

**HEALING CODES:** Do the Healing Codes exercise on page 189 in *Perfect Weight America*. Record your stress level as you rated it while doing the exercise.

| Healing Codes (AM) | Beginning: | End: | 10 min. later: |
|---|---|---|---|
| Healing Codes (PM) | Beginning: | End: | 10 min. later: |

Did you meet your Phase IV goals today? _____

Record your thoughts, insights, and questions; your emotional outlook and physical state; and your successes and challenges.

_____

_____

_____

**Record everything you consume, including food, snacks, supplements, water, mints, and gum.**

**Breakfast**

Water:
Supplements:
Morning snack:

**Lunch**

Water:
Supplements:
Midday snack:

**Dinner**

Water:
Supplements:
Evening snack:

**Exercise**

**HEALING CODES: Do the Healing Codes exercise on page 189 in *Perfect Weight America*. Record your stress level as you rated it while doing the exercise.**

| Healing Codes (AM) | Beginning: | End: | 10 min. later: |
| Healing Codes (PM) | Beginning: | End: | 10 min. later: |

Did you meet your Phase IV goals today? _____

Record your thoughts, insights, and questions; your emotional outlook and physical state; and your successes and challenges.

_____

_____

_____

# Summary of Week 16

How many days did you follow the Perfect Weight Eating Plan? _____

How many days did you take the recommended supplements? _____

How many days did you drink at least half your body weight in ounces of water?

_____

How many days did you meet your goals for Phase IV? _____

How many days did you exercise this week? _____

Write down any extra thoughts you want to capture about your week.

_____

_____

_____

_____

_____

_____

_____

_____

_____

_____

_____

_____

_____

_____

_____

# Personal Thoughts

## Personal Thoughts

## Personal Thoughts

## Personal Thoughts